ADD & ROMANCE

*Finding Fulfillment in Love,
Sex, & Relationships*

Jonathan Scott Halverstadt, M.S.

TAYLOR TRADE PUBLISHING
Lanham • New York • Oxford

For my loving wife, Terri
143, 2 — 4 ∞

Book design by Mark McGarry
Set in Goudy

Published by Taylor Trade Publishing
An Imprint of the Rowman & Littlefield Publishing Group
4501 Forbes Blvd., Suite 200
Lanham, Maryland 20706

Distributed by National Book Network

Library of Congress Cataloging-in-Publication Data

Halverstadt, Jonathan Scott.
    ADD & romance : finding fulfillment in love, sex & relationships /
Jonathan Scott Halverstadt.
        p.   cm.
    ISBN 0-87833-209-X
    1. Man-woman relationships.   2. Attention-deficit disordered adults.
I. Title.
HQ801.H3225   1998
306.7—dc21   98-39387
                                                  CIP

Printed in the United States of America

Contents

Foreword

Jonathan Scott Halverstadt and I have worked together as a team at my clinic for the last several years. We have worked with hundreds of children, teenagers, and adults who have been suffering from the behavioral symptoms caused by Attention Deficit Disorder. And with his deep understanding of ADD, Jonathan has been able to help those patients cope with their difficulties and learn how to lead positive, exciting lives.

As someone who has struggled with this disorder his whole life, Jonathan understands ADD on an intensely personal level. He understands the joy his patients feel from effective treatment. And he understands their brand-new sense of hope for the future.

But Jonathan doesn't just bring his personal experience to the treatment of ADD. He also brings an understanding of the neurobiology of this disorder and extensive experience studying the ADD brain in action using nuclear brain imaging techniques.

Jonathan brings both the reality of living with ADD and the science of this disorder together in *ADD & Romance*. In a balanced approach, Jonathan highlights the strengths of people with ADD and the struggles that cause them and their partners pain. If you or your partners suffer from ADD and you've been wondering why your romantic relationships just don't work out, this book will clarify your problems and provide solutions that really work. There is hope—here are answers.

When it comes to ADD and romance, Jonathan Scott Halverstadt knows what works, both through his own personal experiences and those of his hundreds of patients. *ADD & Romance* brings it all together for you. You *can* have the relationship of your dreams.

Daniel G. Amen, M.D.
Director, The Amen Clinic for Behavioral Medicine
Fairfield, California

Acknowledgments

First and foremost I want to thank my wife, Terri, who has been a constant source of help and encouragement with this project and in my life. If the reader finds any encouragement or solace in these pages, it is partly due to Terri's encouragement and understanding over the many months it took me to write this.

I would also like to thank the following people for their help and encouragement: My parents, Lee and Dorothy Halverstadt, for holding my hand and my heart when I was hurting the most, and, for the love you have always had for me, even through all those tough years; Daniel G. Amen, M.D., for the impact you have had upon the world through your research, and especially for the impact you have had upon my life—God is using you in a mighty way and I am thankful that I have the opportunity to work with you as a colleague on a daily basis; my agent, Mary Brice, for believing in me and in this project; my editor and coach, Janis Leibs Dworkis, for her genuine interest and many hours of work; Camille Cline, Stacey Sexton, and Stephanie Milacek at Taylor Publishing for their help, patience, and expertise; my colleagues at the Amen Clinic; and my friends: the Brucemeister, Greg and Donna Brock, Dwight and Pat Dalton, John Howard, Matthew Stubblefield, Wendy Richardson, Marilyn Watts, Brian Goldman, Carolyn Trace, Bart Gibson, Earl Henslin, Keith and Andrea Miller, Les

Lucas, Dwaine McCallon, Lynn Weiss, Jerry Seiden, Ali and Clyde Baker, John and Reva McKie, John and Karen Fu, Rich Scileppi, Ric Seaberg, Sterg, Jim Moore, Lesli Pepper, Pamela Powell, Jack and Dorothy Vance, Tony Yamamoto, and the Thursday Night Fun Club. You have all had a part in this book in one way or another because you have all contributed so richly to my life. Thank you. Maranatha!

Introduction

Attention Deficit Disorder (ADD) affects every aspect of a person's life. Most people who have it were born with it—and it never goes away. You carry it with you your whole life. For better or worse, it influences almost everything you do.

I know exactly how ADD affects a person's life, because I have it myself.

I never knew I had ADD until I was in my late thirties. I was working as a therapist, having just received my master's degree in marriage and family counseling, and I was at a conference on learning disabilities and ADD. In every session I attended, I was amazed—because they were discussing my life. They were discussing the difficulties I had always had academically. They were discussing the difficulties I had at work. And they were discussing the difficulties I had in my interpersonal relationships.

That's when I realized I needed to see someone who could give me a professional diagnosis. And when I did that, the diagnosis was ADD.

Looking back on my life from that point, with that diagnosis in hand, I was able to see that ADD had brought a lot of positive attributes into my life. My sensitivity and intuition are ADD traits, traits that help me greatly in my work. And ADD has allowed me to study and learn many different types of information at one time, and to do many activities at one time. Before I turned thirty, for example, I had already written my first book, earned my private pilot's license, worked as a network announcer for NBC and CBS TV, been a ski instructor, written and produced award-winning advertising campaigns, performed in thousands of radio and TV commercials, been an executive editor of a magazine published in five languages, and had a re-occurring role on *General Hospital*. And I owe my ability to have accomplished so many things at one time to my ADD.

But I could also see the difficulties ADD had brought into my life. I had always had academic problems, and in high school I had become despondent about them. Everyone around me told me I could do the work if I would just try harder. But I was trying as hard as I possibly could, and I was flunking two of my classes. In my personal relationships, I would say things impulsively—things that were better left unsaid. I tried to pay attention to my partner, but I wasn't really focused, I wasn't really all there. In fact, I believe that the demise of my first marriage was due in great part to my undiagnosed and untreated ADD.

Now, after working with ADD clients as a therapist for years, I have come to believe that undiagnosed and untreated ADD is one of the major causes of divorce in this country.

And that is the reason I have written this book. So many couples have difficulty in their relationships because one or both of the partners has undiagnosed and untreated ADD as the underlying problem. All too often, their ADD goes undetected even though they may have spent a considerable amount of time in therapy working to improve their relationship. Without an accurate diagnosis, people can try and try to "get better" without fully attaining the results they work so hard to achieve—just like I tried and tried to do better in school but still failed classes. If you have ADD, you need a diagnosis and treatment before you can break through that barrier.

Introduction

What we know about ADD is that it is a medical problem and needs to be treated medically. Medicine is not magic. Even with medication you'll still have to work at changing old behaviors and old patterns of relating to others, but it is certainly easier to overcome those difficulties with the help of medication.

In the first part of the book, we are going to discuss the difficulties that ADD brings to relationships, and it's important to get that information out there. But don't become bogged down by the negatives. Because if you stick with the book, you'll see the positives, too.

I have been treated for ADD for several years now, and it has definitely turned my life around. I have a wonderful marriage. I have better impulse control. I have choices available to me that weren't available before my ADD was under control. Now I can choose what I do, and I can make choices that are best for my family and for my life.

Now I know my future is full of hope. And I know yours can be, too. That's what *ADD & Romance* is all about.

JONATHAN SCOTT HALVERSTADT, M.S.

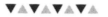

ONE

The Effects of ADD on Romantic Relationships—One Couple's Story

Come meet some friends of mine, Annie and Bob Wilson. I love these people dearly. And they love each other dearly, too. Unfortunately, they drive each other nuts. And they drive everyone else around them nuts, too.

You have never met more argumentative and impulsive people in your life. You've never seen a home that was a bigger mess. And the truth is that their lives are as disorganized as their home. They have been late to every date we've ever planned together, except for the ones they've forgotten altogether, and their poor kids have been stranded at school more often than they care to remember.

Annie and Bob met in college at a party thrown by a mutual friend. As they tell it, it was love at first sight.

Annie was immediately impressed by Bob's hobbies. "He was a skydiver. And that was something I had always wanted to do. All that night, I kept asking him what it felt like to be falling straight toward the earth. I hung onto his every word as he described to me what a rush it was. I just kept imagining that feeling over and over again. I knew I wanted to feel that for myself."

Bob couldn't believe his great luck, and he took Annie out to a skydiving school the very next day. The adrenaline and endorphin

5

rushes were the best the two of them had ever felt. The chemistry was perfect. They were a match made in heaven, or so they thought.

From then on, they were inseparable. Bob called her apartment four times a day. He sent flowers and teddy bears and singing telegrams. Annie, who had never been courted like this before, decided that this is what it must feel like to really be in love. She craved and loved the attention. She cooked for Bob. She did his laundry. She baked him cookies almost every day. She mailed him love notes.

They knew they were right for each other. Neither had ever been this happy before. So on the spur of the moment, while driving back to school, they took a little side trip and got married. They had never been happier.

When they got back to Annie's apartment, they notified Annie's roommate that she would be moving out, because Bob would be moving in. And they began to set up their first home together.

When Annie looked at Bob's furniture in her apartment, she decided they needed some new things. Bob suggested they wait to buy furniture until he graduated the following month and had income from a job he had already been offered. But Annie said, "Why should we wait? You graduate next month. You'll be working. We'll have money. What's to worry about?"

So while Bob was in school later that first week, Annie got a friend to help her pull Bob's old couch outside for Goodwill to pick up. Then she went out and bought two reclining chairs and an antique end table.

"Of course, I also got a few other little things," Annie says. "Some lamps, new dishes and glassware, and some beautiful new towels. You can't expect to start a marriage off without new towels, can you? Everyone has to have them."

But when Bob came home, he saw things differently. His favorite, most comfortable couch was gone. And in its place was an enormous credit card bill that neither of them had the money to pay. They suddenly owed $2,500 more than they had owed the day before. And he was furious.

"How could you do this!" he screamed at Annie. "What are you? Stupid? Don't you know that we don't have this kind of money? How are we going to pay for all this stuff? And we didn't even need it anyway!"

"Yes we did!" Annie screamed back at him. "Are you too stupid to know what it takes to set up an apartment? You can't just live with hand-me-down furniture forever. And anyway, you'll be starting your job soon. Everything will be okay."

"Who's the one who's stupid here?" Bob yelled. And he stormed out of the house. Annie went to bed alone and crying. She sobbed into her pillow, realizing that she had made a terrible mistake by marrying this man.

But when Bob came back an hour later, he was carrying flowers. "I'm so sorry," he said. "I never meant to hurt you. We'll figure out how to pay for this somehow. Don't worry." And they made up and made mad, passionate love.

The next day, the mail brought the answer to their problems. Annie saw it before Bob got home. It was an offer for a new credit card. And when she filled out the application, Annie realized it would solve everything. They could use this new credit card to pay off the old one! Everything would be fine.

And that's how it was for Annie and Bob in those early years. They would fight and scream and yell, and then realize they both wanted to make up. They would both spend too much money on things they didn't really need. They would each say terribly hurtful things to the other, and then apologize the next day and say again how much they loved each other. They knew they spent a lot of time being unhappy. But they also knew they loved each other. It was a very intense relationship. As if that were not enough, children were added to their lives and life got even more intense.

The first time I was in Annie and Bob's house, I was speechless. This was their second home since their initial apartment. It was a big, beautiful two-story home with the kids' rooms upstairs and a huge backyard. But what made my mouth hang open were the piles of clutter on absolutely every single surface in this home. Bob, who often brought work home from the office, had piles of work papers everywhere throughout the house—including on his bathroom sink. And Annie had piles of her work papers on every surface of the kitchen, including the stove top.

There were kids' toys and dog toys covering the floor of every room. The kitchen pantry was open and potatoes were literally rolling out onto the floor. Bills and checks were piled high on a small table in the corner of the kitchen. And a big wooden crate sat in the very middle of the living room, making it almost impossible to walk through the room.

"I'm in the middle of building some furniture," Bob said about the living room. "I've been working on it for quite a while. This is going to be a living room table. And this over here is going to be a video cabinet and a bookcase for my daughter's room. I hope to have it finished by Christmas."

Annie chimed in from the kitchen. "He always says that . . . he just never says Christmas of which year! He's been saying that since two Christmases ago."

The dining room table was covered with Annie's unfinished sewing projects and an electric drill and drill bits. "My sewing machine wasn't working real well. I decided that I could service it myself," Annie said. "But I don't know. I just couldn't quite get it right."

When I met Annie and Bob, they had been married for about ten years. They fought constantly about money, their house, their relatives, their children, their cars, and the weather. There were times when I thought that if Annie said it was partly cloudy, Bob would say no, it was partly sunny. In our group of friends, we decided that they must like it that way. They must just love the conflict and arguing.

But when Annie and Bob were getting along, they were the most fun company you could imagine. And that's why they had so many friends. They had more energy and spontaneity than any of us. One time, we all drove twenty-five miles out in the desert to look at the stars at one o'clock in the morning. They just piled their sleeping kids into the van along with us, and we all took off. And another time, we all went white-water rafting together. It was the experience of a lifetime. Bob works part-time on the weekends as a white-water raft instructor, so he knew the river well. Leave it to Annie and Bob to come up with the most wonderfully wild and wacky weekend experiences for the rest of us.

Of course, those were the good times. But then again . . . most of the time, we just wondered why Annie and Bob even stayed together. They seemed to have such an intensity. Positive intensity and negative intensity. There didn't seem to be any middle ground.

And to add to the Wilsons' problems, their son and daughter were having trouble in school. Robby absolutely could not sit still through one single class period. And he couldn't seem to keep quiet, either. He would jump up and talk to his friends right in the middle of class. He would argue with the students on the playground. He would even argue with the teachers. He brought home detention slips for behavior problems every single week. Annie and Bob knew he was intelligent, but he earned very poor grades.

They were very disappointed, but not really surprised, when the principal asked them to come to school for a meeting. They talked and argued for days about what the purpose of the meeting could be. But when the day came, both Annie and Bob forgot to show up, even though it was written on their calendar—even though they both left for work with a yellow sticky note in their pockets as well as on the dash of their cars. They had both simply gotten busy at work and forgotten about the meeting. Robby sat alone in the principal's office, thinking that his parents were too embarrassed by him to even come to the meeting.

Caroline, their daughter, seemed to have a problem that was the opposite of Robby's. Caroline never said anything much at all. In fact, she hardly ever moved at all. Caroline was a daydreamer. She seemed to be perfectly happy to sit for hours at a time and just stare out the window. That was fine if she wanted to "space out" on the weekends, but it didn't work as well in school. Annie and Bob would help her study for a test, for example, and know for a fact that she knew her material perfectly. Then she would bring home a "D" on the test. Why? Because she had started daydreaming in the middle of the test, and never answered more than the first four questions.

What had gone wrong with this family? Why had everything seemed so rosy and then just collapsed?

Annie and Bob really have a problem, and it's a problem that has caused their lives to become more and more chaotic and out of control. Annie and Bob both have Attention Deficit Disorder (ADD), a neurobiological problem in the brain. And contrary to what you might have heard in the popular media, ADD is probably the most *under-diagnosed* psychiatric disorder in this country. It is the cause of millions of unhappy marriages and millions of divorces. The truth? Annie and Bob really do love each other. But unless their problem is properly diagnosed and treated, there really isn't much long-term hope for them. And since both their children also have ADD, there isn't much hope for them either without proper treatment.

Let's look at the specific ways in which ADD is undermining the Wilsons' marriage. The following behaviors are some of those that are typical of people with ADD, and they certainly play a major role in the Wilsons' continual frustration and unhappiness:

1. **Impulsivity.** Why did Annie and Bob get married after only knowing each other for four weeks? Because their ADD left them with little impulse control. They weren't able to think through the consequences of their actions and the options

that might have been available to them. Their brains wouldn't let them.

2. **Need for stimulation.** People with ADD are constantly seeking ways to stimulate their brains. One way they do that early in a romantic relationship is by lavishing attention on people they love. The love notes, the constant phone calls, the flowers, the poetry, the hyperfocusing on each other—all of those are signs of ADD behaviors. But here's the problem: When those actions are no longer stimulating to the person engaging in them, the romancing stops. And the romantic partner can be left wondering what happened. Similarly, projects that initially seem very exciting quickly lose their luster when they are no longer stimulating. And they are likely to be left unfinished.

   Consider Bob's occupation as a fireman and his weekend hobbies of skydiving and white-water rafting. Or Annie, who now also skydives and works full-time as a physician's assistant in the emergency room of a major metropolitan hospital. All very stimulating.

3. **Conflict-seeking behavior.** Often, one of the ways people with ADD stimulate themselves is by arguing. For many of us, arguing is a behavior that doesn't feel good, so we avoid it. But some people with ADD argue a lot because it provides a kind of stimulation for their brain. So they may seek that stimulation, usually subconsciously, by provoking arguments.

4. **Forgetfulness.** People with ADD forget things all the time, no matter how important those things are—from appointments, to where they put things, to people's names. They just simply forget. Annie and Bob both had every intention of making that meeting with Robby's principal. They certainly understood how important it was. But they forgot. Annie and Bob even tried marital counseling for a few sessions, but kept forgetting their appointments.

5. **Poor communication skills.** Good communication requires good listening and good verbalization skills. People with ADD often have neither. That's because their brains are racing ahead to the next thought, or, like Caroline, off in a fantasy world altogether unrelated to the conversation at hand. And poor communication always hurts a relationship.

6. **Lack of organization.** The piles of laundry and paperwork, the misplaced keys, and the lifestyle that appears to be in complete disarray are all hallmarks of ADD. It's hard to be organized when your brain is either running at a million miles a minute or daydreaming. Add to that all the uncompleted tasks that the individual has every intention of completing but has been unable to complete because of distraction after distraction. Due to that inability to stay on task, nothing gets completed and things pile up.

Sounds pretty hopeless, doesn't it? But the most important thing I want you to know is this: *This problem can usually be fixed.* ADD is a medical problem. And it is a medical problem for which we now have many effective medical treatments.

So, in Chapter Two, we're going to talk about the causes of ADD and what can be done medically to treat it. Because the sooner we fix the problem, the better things will be for you.

Mind you, having ADD isn't all bad. There are some wonderful things about having ADD that make life a whole lot better for everyone. Yes—there are gifts that come along with ADD. Annie is a wonderful emergency room physician's assistant partly because of her ADD. The same is true for Bob in his occupations as fireman and white-water rafting guide. But we'll take a look at the positive things ADD has to contribute to life and relationships later on, in Chapter Seven. For now, let's take a closer look at what ADD really is and at some of the things that can be done about its negative aspects.

▼▲▼▲▼▲▼

TWO

▲▼▲▼▲▼▼

"I Thought Only Kids Got That"

If you knew much about ADD before reading this book, chances are you've heard about ADD in reference to children. You've heard about the little boy who just cannot stay in his seat at school. He squirms, he wiggles, he bangs his legs against the chair. Or the little girl who's great on the soccer field—but has trouble with her schoolwork, talks constantly in class, and can't seem to stop herself from sassing her teacher. Or the boy who doesn't have any outward behavior problems at all, but consistently performs significantly below his potential.

What you might not know is that ADD is a part of those children's lives forever, into and through adulthood. ADD is not a childhood problem that just mysteriously disappears during adolescence. But that's what therapists and physicians thought for many years. Some, who are not current with the most recent research, still believe that today.

In truth, ADD is a medical disorder, and current research indicates that a person who is born with ADD will most likely have that disorder for his or her entire life. More specifically, ADD is a neurobiological problem. That means it is a problem caused by a malfunction in the brain. In other words, the causes of ADD are physical.

The first thing we need to do, in order to begin to understand ADD, is take a quick look at the brain and how it works.

The brain is an information processing center. Information constantly comes into the brain from every part of the body, and the brain constantly sends information back out. The cells that carry that information are called nerve cells, or neurons.

Imagine the pathway of the nervous system as millions and millions of neurons all lined up in a row. Each cell passes information—in the form of an electrical impulse—to the next, and that cell passes it on to the next, etc. It's similar to a line of people passing sandbags or buckets of water from one to the next. But the crucial difference between the line of neurons in the nervous system and the line of people passing sandbags is that the neurons can't quite touch each other.

Between each neuron and the next is a gap about a millionth of an inch wide. That gap, called a synapse, might not sound like much, but it is wide enough to keep one cell from passing along its information to the next. It's as if the people passing the sandbags were each standing fifteen feet apart. You just aren't going to get those sandbags very far down the line that way.

In the central nervous system, the brain produces specific chemicals to help information cross those millions of synapses. Those chemicals are called neurotransmitters. Neurotransmitters act as chemical bridges that allow information to flow from one neuron to the next, to the next, to the next . . . and so on.

When you have the right kind of neurotransmitter available at the right time in the right place in the right amount, your nervous system just kind of hums along and you're in great shape. But if the biochemistry isn't right, your internal information processing system can decrease in effectiveness, and that can negatively affect your behavior.

And that's exactly what causes ADD. ADD has nothing to do with a person's willful misbehavior. It has everything to do with a person's neurobiological deficit. That deficit can be inherited genetically, or it can result from head trauma. But in any case, that deficit is most likely with the person for life. Symptoms may change in their expression from childhood to adulthood, and compensating skills may hide the symptoms, but the neurobiology is the same. Fortunately, ADD can be treated medically so that the symptoms either lessen or practically disappear. But the underlying cause of those ADD symptoms never goes away.

The particular part of the brain that causes ADD symptoms is the prefrontal cortex, located at the front of the brain directly behind the forehead. This is the part of the brain that is responsible for "executive functioning."

When all goes well, the prefrontal cortex helps you run your life just like an effective CEO runs a successful corporation. You take in information from various sources, process the information carefully in the prefrontal cortex, and make behavioral decisions that will best help you meet your short-term and long-term goals.

For example, suppose you're a CEO of a large corporation and you have to make a decision about whether or not to sell 100,000 units of a commodity at a given price. You couldn't make that decision in a vacuum. You'd need to have information about supply, demand, cost, international markets, etc. You'd find that information by using your telephone and computer modem to connect with your associates around the world and throughout your company.

But if the phone lines or the computer networks were down, you wouldn't be able to access the information you need to make good decisions for the corporation. And that's exactly what people with ADD have to deal with in their brain. The computer is there—the best computer ever created—but the phone lines are down. And no matter how wonderful the computer is, it can't process information it isn't getting—or getting fast enough.

When the information system of your prefrontal cortex isn't working well—when the electrical impulses aren't flowing properly—you lose some of your capacity to clearly understand the information coming in to you. You lose your ability to process that information in the context of your personal goals and make behavioral decisions that are in your best interest. Instead, you misinterpret social and physical cues, you jump to conclusions without thinking things through, you act impulsively without concern for consequences, and you lose your ability to stay focused on your long-term goals.

In other words, when the electrical activity in your prefrontal cortex is sluggish because of a lack of the appropriate neurotransmitter, called dopamine, you exhibit the behaviors we call ADD.

I want to repeat this because it is so important, so crucial: ADD is the result of an underactive prefrontal cortex. And that underactivity results from an inadequate supply of a neurotransmitter called dopamine.

As you now see, ADD is a set of behaviors that results from a neurobiological disorder. It is not a set of behaviors that results from a desire to undermine relationships, or a desire to be selfish, or a desire to disrupt family life. ADD results from a physical disorder. And similar to arthritis, or muscular dystrophy, or epilepsy, ADD is no one's fault.

The Types of ADD

Although ADD has been around for a long time, it hasn't always been called ADD. In the past, it's been called "Organic Drivenness," "Minimal Brain Dysfunction," and "Hyperkinetic," to name a few. Today, physicians, therapists, and others who treat people with ADD know the disorder by its by more technical name, ADHD—Attention Deficit Hyperactivity Disorder. But because ADD is the term most commonly used by the layperson, we will be using the terms ADD and ADHD interchangeably in this book.

Not everyone with an underactive prefrontal cortex exhibits the same set of ADD symptoms. In fact, three specific types of ADD (or ADHD) have been identified. They are:

- **ADHD predominantly hyperactive/impulsive type.** This is the type of ADD in which the predominant characteristics are hyperactivity (often experienced as restlessness in adults) and impulsivity. People with this type of ADD are often attracted to intense physical and/or mental activities and professions such as emergency room doctor, firefighter, or comedian.
- **ADHD predominantly inattentive type.** This is the type of ADD in which the predominant characteristics are inconsistency in attention, apparent lack of motivation, and daydreaming. People with this type of ADD generally do not exhibit hyperactivity.
- **ADHD combined type.** This is the type of ADD in which the predominant characteristics are a combination of the previous two types.

Some people who have ADD also have abnormal activity levels in another part, or parts, of their brain. In particular, there are people who suffer from decreased activity in their prefrontal cortex combined with increased activity of their cingulate gyrus (*sing-u-lat ji-rus*).

The cingulate gyrus (also called simply "the cingulate") is located in an area of the brain that starts at the top of the head and comes down over the top of the brain all the way down into the prefrontal cortex. When the cingulate is overactive, people tend to "get stuck" in their thinking. They may worry a lot. They may have difficulty shifting gears from one subject to another, and difficulty seeing options in a situation once they have their mind set on something. They tend to hold onto their own opinions and not listen to others. They seem to be stubborn and argumentative.

This particular combination of decreased prefrontal cortex

activity along with increased cingulate activity, and the behaviors that result from it, were first identified by Daniel G. Amen, M.D., at the clinic where I work in California—the Amen Clinic for Behavioral Medicine. About 800 patients from around the world come to the clinic every month, and we've seen a total of about 50,000 patients in the last eight years, more than 8,000 of whom have had ADD. By working with this vast number of patients, and by studying many of their brains via nuclear brain imaging, Dr. Amen identified this particular prefrontal cortex/cingulate pattern. We call this condition the "overfocused" subtype of ADD.

The exact group of behaviors caused by this overfocused subtype depends on what type of ADD the person has. For example, one person could have ADHD predominantly hyperactive/impulsive type along with the overfocused subtype, and someone else could have ADHD predominantly inattentive type along with the over-focused subtype. So, the overfocused subtype can co-exist with various types of ADD.

What Does ADD Look Like?

What does ADD look like in adults? Depending on the lifestyle the adult has chosen, ADD can look much like it did for the child in the classroom. If the adult with ADD has taken a job that forces him to sit still behind a desk all day, he might find himself getting up and down, restless and unable to stay still. Or if she has taken a job that requires extensive reading and paperwork, she might feel discouraged because she is always behind in her work. But if the adult with ADD works as a football coach, or as an emergency room doctor or nurse, a psychotherapist, or an artist, you might not see any ADD symptoms on the job. In fact, certain ADD traits can be an asset in some of those professions.

Regardless of the job an ADD adult has chosen, ADD traits will most likely emerge in his or her romantic relationships. And if you don't have ADD but are involved with an ADD partner, it can be very frustrating. Or if *you* are the ADD partner, and you don't understand why the relationship is so difficult for you, the frustration level can be equally high. Thousands of ADD men and women have spent years in therapy to try to work out their relationship problems so they can have a more satisfying life, but find many of the changes they had hoped for eluded them. Why didn't all those years in therapy and thousands of dollars pay off? Because at the heart of their problems was this frustrating disorder which was believed to have only been present in little boys, something only male children were diagnosed with.

Here's what ADD can look like in romantic relationships. As you read through this list, think about how many of these behaviors apply to your own relationships.

1) "He just isn't really there for me." (Not fully present emotionally and/or intellectually.)

Sarah and Richard have been dating for three years and are engaged to be married next spring. At the beginning of their relationship, Richard lavished more attention on Sarah than she had ever experienced in her life. He called her every day and seemed to hang on every word she said. She felt she was important to Richard—the most important thing in his life.

But lately, Sarah has begun to worry. Richard still calls her every day, and they see each other very often. But when they are together, Sarah has a vague feeling that Richard isn't really paying attention to her. He just doesn't seem to be completely present with her. When they're talking about plans for their future home, Richard will nod his head and contribute to the conversation every now and then, but his heart and his mind just don't seem to be into it. And when Sarah looks into Richard's eyes, she isn't sure what she's seeing. He seems distant. She wonders if his love for her is waning.

He doesn't seem to care for her like he did when they were first dating. On the other hand, Richard is totally in love with Sarah and assures her of that regularly. Richard has never loved anyone as deeply as Sarah. He loves her with all of his heart and truly wants Sarah to be his lifelong partner. Yet Sarah doesn't feel the love that Richard has for her.

What's bothering Sarah, what makes her feel as if Richard doesn't really care for her, is that although Richard himself is physically present, his ADD mind isn't always completely there with her. Sarah is picking up on that subtlety, and she is interpreting it correctly: Richard isn't always completely present with her—emotionally or mentally. But what Sarah might be misinterpreting is the reason behind that distance. While Sarah might worry that Richard doesn't really love her the way he used to, Richard's love for Sarah might have been growing all along. His heart is with her 100 percent, but his ADD mind is not.

This distance exists because a person with ADD often has many, many different thoughts going on at one time—with virtually no control over that scattered thinking process. For example, Sarah might talk to Richard about golfing lessons, and Richard might be genuinely interested. But while he's listening to her talk about her lessons, he's also thinking about the report he has due at work, his dog who needs to be fed, the way the sunlight is striking Sarah's face at that exact moment, the weather forecast he heard on the way to work, his brother's birthday, the pants he needs to take to the cleaners, his new neighbor's cat, the basketball game he was in last week . . . And all the while, he's nodding at Sarah and answering her questions. He can even sometimes listen well enough to paraphrase back to her what she said and still not be fully present in the conversation because of his multi-tasking mind.

Richard is genuinely interested in what Sarah is saying. But what she's picking up on is that his mind is partly somewhere else. Sarah is left to wonder and feel hurt because she doesn't know about

ADD. She often feels alone even when Richard is physically present. It's one thing to be alone. It's another thing completely—the most painful kind of alone—to be alone when you are with the person you love.

Because the ADD partner is often not completely present when he is with his partner, it's pretty common for the non-ADD partner to think the other person doesn't love them anymore. In contrast, the ADD partner might care about his mate totally and completely. But that fact isn't coming across. Unfortunately, the non-ADD partner becomes more and more lonely in the relationship. Sarah needs to learn about ADD and it's effect on romantic relationships. Otherwise, she may decide to leave the relationship because she doesn't get that he loves her.

2) "She doesn't think before she acts or speaks." (Impulsiveness.)

Matthew and Toni have been married for seventeen years, and their two children are teenagers now. Both boys are good students and good drivers. They manage their budgets well, make good decisions about friends, and are generally very responsible. Matthew is thrilled that his teens are doing so well. He wishes his wife were in such good shape. Her behavior strikes him as more adolescent than their adolescents' behavior. In a way, it's like that in conversations too.

"If Toni's thinking, she's speaking," Matthew says.

It frustrates him that Toni seems to be in her own little world, oblivious to the normal ebb and flow of conversation. It doesn't matter what the topic of conversation is or how much Toni has already monopolized the discussion, she butts in and starts speaking. And for some reason, she doesn't seem to pick up on the fact that she's interrupting anyone—or that they might not be the least bit interested in what she has to say. Toni's friends usually put up with it, but Matthew finds her habits very frustrating and hurtful. No matter what he tries to express to Toni, he doesn't seem to be important enough to her to not interrupt him. She might say that she cares about what he's saying, but she obviously doesn't care enough to really listen. She's tried to work on her interrupting problem and has gotten as far as butting in with phrases like, "Excuse me," or, "May I interrupt for a moment?" These are really only polite ways of being impolite. It seems impossible for Matthew to begin to communicate something without Toni politely interrupting his train of thought with some disjointed comment and then channeling the conversation in a completely different direction (if not some completely different topic). Talk about frustrating.

Some days, Matthew wonders if there's any point in trying to talk to Toni at all. Why bother trying to share his thoughts or his feelings when she's clearly not interested in what he has to say?

What is bothering Matthew in his relationship with Toni is her impulsive behavior, one of the key symptoms of the hyperactive/impulsive form of ADD. And when it comes to relationships, two of the main problem areas caused by impulsivity are communication and finances.

Toni has ADHD predominantly hyperactive/impulsive type. If she sees it and she's attracted to it, out of her impulsiveness (caused by lack of stimulation in the prefrontal cortex part of her brain) she reaches out and the next thing she knows, she's bought a brand-new pair of earrings. Or an unusual pair of shoes. Or a new shade of lipstick. All she knows is that she wants it. She doesn't stop to think about how much the item will cost or whether she already has one almost exactly like it. She just wants it, and so she buy it. Because she has ADD, her brain isn't putting on the brakes, so to speak—suggesting that she take a minute to re-evaluate her purchase. So she barrels right along. The same way she does in conversations.

Toni shops at many of the finer department stores because of their generous return policies. She may even have more personal contact with the customer relations people at the return counter at Nordstroms than she does with some of her colleagues at work. Her impulsive buying drives Matthew nuts. But he doesn't even know about a lot of the impulsive purchases she makes because often, by the time she gets home, she realizes she made an impulsive purchase and takes it back before he even sees it. On occasion, Toni will buy something during her lunch hour as she walks by a kiosk with merchandise that seems to be screaming "Buy me!" to her. Then she'll return it on her way home. This is not fun for either her or Matthew. It's a real sore spot in their relationship.

I do want to differentiate Toni's ADD-related *impulsive* spending from the *compulsive* spending that afflicts people with other brain disorders. Toni is an *impulsive* shopper who spends money because she sees something she wants and doesn't stop to think of the consequences of purchasing it. Her purchases aren't necessarily extravagant or expensive, they're just constant and often unnecessary.

People who are *compulsive* shoppers have an addictive need that cannot be satisfied by any activity other than shopping, and their purchases often are extravagant. Compulsive shoppers will leave their houses on a shopping binge with the goal of buying something, because shopping and spending are the only activities that alleviate their states of anxiety. True, they may spend *impulsively*, but it is the compulsion to spend that drives them. Toni probably leaves her house every day with something else entirely on her mind. In fact, she may leave for the grocery store repeating aloud to herself while driving in her car, "I'm only going to buy milk, butter, and eggs. Matt needs me to stay on track with our budget." But by the time she returns home, she has $150 worth of groceries—most of which were on sale, most of which the family will be able to use . . . sometime. Her rationale is that she really was saving the family money in the long run because of the money saved through sale items. Although her plan to save the family money was great, there is a huge difference between a $10 purchase and a $150 purchase.

In this particular scenario, the mortgage payment was a little short that month because of her impulsive spending. Not to mention that she even forgot to get the eggs, one of the three items she originally went to the market to purchase.

Matthew remembers the day Toni pointed out the balding spot on the back of his head. "Hey, honey, looks like you're going bald," she said, the very second she noticed the spot. It's just hair, he rationalized to himself, and he knew he wasn't as young as he used to be. But Toni's comment was painful for him. Why hadn't she realized that would hurt his feelings? "Maybe she just didn't care," Matthew thought.

Actually, Toni does care about Matthew's feelings. But she hadn't realized her comment would be hurtful because, just like her shopping experiences, her brain hadn't applied the brakes. She didn't have the ability to think it through. The thought was there, and she spoke it impulsively. That's also why Toni monopolizes conversations and interrupts when others are talking. Her untreated ADD doesn't give her a chance to consider the consequences of her actions. In retrospect, she is usually able to see where and how she was being impulsive, and she can tell you what behaviors would have been more appropriate and productive for the relationship. But like the grocery shopping scenario above, in the moment when the impulsive behaviors are happening, she just doesn't have the insight or control she needs to be more appropriate.

Unfortunately for her marriage, the consequences of those actions are often quite hurtful.

3) "He'd forget his own head if it wasn't screwed on tight." (Forgetful.)

Donald met Megan six years ago during their freshman year in college and has been completely in love with her ever since. She is the most beautiful woman he has ever seen. She is warm, lively, caring—everything he has ever wanted. Two months ago, Donald asked Megan to marry him. To his terrible surprise, she said she wasn't really sure she was ready to take that step of "until death do us part." She assured him that she loved him and that there was no one else in her life, but she said his behavior was just too irresponsible. She wasn't sure she could count on him.

Donald was stunned. Looking back over the previous six years, he felt he had done absolutely everything for this woman he could imagine. He took her out, he wrote her love notes, he nursed her back to health when she was sick. He even helped her brother move into a new apartment in the next town. What more could he have done to show his love? How much more responsible could he have been?

Plenty, according to Megan.

Yes, Donald has done many wonderful and romantic things over the years. But all too often, he did not come through when he said he would. He'd make plans for a wonderful romantic dinner, plan everything just so—and then be an hour and a half late to pick Megan up. While she was waiting and fuming, Donald was talking for an hour to an old friend he ran into at the gas station. Then there was the time on a Friday that he promised her he would pick her up right after work because her car was in the shop. He showed up an hour late—too late for her to get her car out of the shop until Monday. Where had he been while Megan waited outside in the dark? He had been listening to music with his neighbor's son. He'd just left his apartment to get Megan when the kid next door came over and asked if Donald wanted to see his new CD player. Donald thought, "What the heck, that'll only take a couple of minutes." Besides, he didn't want to hurt the kid's feelings. But then he forgot about the time and the next thing he knew, he was running red lights, adrenaline racing through his body, trying to think up an excuse other than "I forgot" or "Honey, I just lost track of time." He knew those excuses had worn thin a long time ago.

If Megan couldn't even count on him to pick her up after work, how could she count on him as a partner to build a life together? "He is a very sweet man and I know he loves me and I love him, but . . ."

Being forgetful is one of the most common ADD traits, and it can easily undermine an otherwise wonderful romantic relationship. When Donald made those plans and commitments, he had every intention of following through. He loves Megan with all his heart and wants her to be a part of his life forever. But as in so many aspects of Donald's life, his intentions and his actions can be two different things.

Usually, it's not that people with ADD actually forget what they had intended to do, although this can happen—it's more that they get sidetracked in the process. But if you get sidetracked too many times when you were planning to pay the electric bill, make the bank deposit, fill that prescription, or pick up your significant other from work, day-to-day life can become pretty miserable.

For example, Donald didn't forget that he had a romantic dinner planned with Megan. But when he stopped to fill up his car and saw his old friend, his brain turned in that new direction. Seeing his old friend was stimulating for him, and he enjoyed that sense of stimulation—as would anyone. But when his brain changed directions on him, he was temporarily sidetracked from his initial plan of action. Unfortunately, that "temporarily" was enough to ruin the evening for Megan, who wondered if Donald had just forgotten their special date altogether. Likewise, when the neighbor's child asked Donald to listen to his new CD player, Donald didn't forget about Megan. But his brain immediately took him in the direction of that new stimulation. Once again, while Donald was doing what he believed was a good thing, Megan was sitting outside, terrified something terrible had happened to him, fuming because here was another time he had let her down, and all the while wondering how she could ever count on this man again.

The kind of behaviors we have been talking about are often labeled by therapists as *passive/aggressive*. This means that the offending partner (in this case, Donald) has unconscious and unexpressed anger towards his partner. Unable to express his anger directly and appropriately through dialogue, his anger is subconsciously expressed in passive ways. Rather than say I am angry with you, his demeanor says "I love you" . . . but his actions are hurtful. It is described as passive/aggressive behavior because it is a camouflaged way of expressing anger, a sneak attack to express anger without ever getting caught.

When ADD is undiagnosed and untreated, people often get labeled as passive/aggressive. Passive/aggressive? Nonsense. Donald's behaviors are not passive/aggressive. This is about ADD, and people who have ADD are forgetful. Give them the right medication at the right dose for their brain and chances are there will be a major decrease in these types of behaviors. Their forgetfulness has to do with a brain that isn't performing the way it was designed to perform, not because they have some ax to grind with their partner and are unable to confront them face to face. Don't get me wrong, it is possible for people with ADD to have passive/aggressive behaviors. The challenge is to be able to identify which behaviors are passive/aggressive and which behaviors are ADD.

People with ADD forget all kinds of stuff. Typically they'll forget important dates, and that's rarely good for a relationship. If you forget your wife's birthday, how happy is she going to be about that? Or if you've forgotten your anniversary three times in the last four years, how many more anniversaries do you think you're going to have? Could be you're treading on thin ice at that point.

Donald, like so many people with ADD, loves his partner dearly. His heart is clearly in the right place. But for Megan's taste, he may have forgotten their appointments, her birthday, and his car payment one too many times. If Donald were treated for his ADD and Megan were educated about his ADD, the relationship would have a much better chance of surviving and thriving. All too often a person's feelings and sense of significance to their partner are dashed against the rocks because they don't really understand what is taking place in their partner's brain neurology.

4) "She never finishes anything she starts." (Poor follow-through.)

Jamie is not a person who sits and watches life pass her by. She is a doer. In fact, she's usually doing ten things at once—sewing, reading several books, volunteering at church, gardening, aerobic dancing, working with the neighborhood watch association, and pet-sitting for friends, just to name a few. Initially, it was exactly this high energy level that attracted Stan. A man fifteen years Jamie's senior, Stan realistically describes himself as a watcher. He enjoys television, movies, and any other activity that doesn't require much physical action. He is just a low-energy kind of guy. When he met Jamie, he was amazed at her energy, her enthusiasm, her willingness to try almost anything. He asked her to marry him a year after they met, and they were married the following month.

But when the honeymoon phase was over, Stan began to notice something about Jamie that he had previously overlooked: She rarely, if ever, finished anything she started. For example, she promised him she would make him a bathrobe. He didn't really need another robe, but he thought it was romantic that she wanted to make it for him. The fact that she never finished it didn't really bother him, but still, he had been looking forward to it.

The reason Jamie hadn't finished making the robe for Stan was that she had become interested in bicycles—not in riding them as much as rebuilding them. She found a great one at a garage sale and decided to refurbish it. Stan thought it sounded like a fun project. But three months later, the bicycle parts were still strewn all over the kitchen table. By that time, Jamie had started and dropped at least ten more projects.

She seldom finished anything. And after a while, it started to really bother Stan. Jamie would start mowing the lawn (he did most of the inside chores, and she did most of the outside chores) but get interrupted and then never quite finish. Stan would offer to finish the lawn, but Jamie would insist that she finish it. But after a while, it would be Stan who had to go outside in the dark to finish that one little 2' x 15' patch of lawn that Jamie never finished mowing. When the kids were little, Jamie would start to plan their birthday parties—but never quite finish sending out the invitations to their friends. And she was always amazed that no one showed up. Days later, Jamie found the unfinished and unsent invitations under a stack of stuff in the bedroom.

Here's a major complaint about poor follow-through. Jamie would start a load of laundry and then, with forty other irons in the fire, become distracted and forget there were damp clothes in the washer. Days later, the clothes were so moldy and musty, the only choice was to throw them away. That can get expensive.

Somehow, Jamie had gone from being a vivacious young woman in Stan's eyes to an immature person flitting from one thing to the next, incapable of finishing anything. To say he was very annoyed is an understatement.

Similar to problems with forgetfulness, people with ADD often find it difficult to finish tasks they have begun. Their heart might be in exactly the right place. They might have every intention of giving their lover a beautiful handmade valentine. But after working on it for thirty minutes and not close to finishing, the ADD partner might get distracted or restless and just leave the card on the table with every intention to come back to it in a few minutes. They might start to balance their checkbook, but not quite finish the task. They might have every intention of tidying up the home, but just never seem to get the clean clothes from the couch back into the closet. Newspapers (many of them never opened) from the last three months have never been taken out to the recycling bin. Bills they paid weeks ago never get to the creditor because even though the checks were written and the envelopes addressed and stamped, none of them were ever mailed.

Jamie is a wonderful woman. Sometimes, even a wonder woman, full of energy and ideas. But she is so easily distracted. Distracted by just about any interruption. Wanting to get everything done but in the process, getting nothing done. Like Jamie, the person with ADD often moves from one task to the next and the next and the next but is unable to complete any of them.

Although the high energy level of people with ADD is often very attractive to a mate, the reality of poor follow-through can become annoying and frustrating very quickly.

5) "Even his piles of papers have piles of papers." (Piles of "stuff.")

Jenny was attracted to Dave from their very first meeting, but she didn't think the relationship could really work. They lived in different cities, six hours apart. They had met at a trade convention. He asked if she would see him again, but she said she didn't think a long-distance relationship was a good idea. Nevertheless, Dave started calling her, and pretty soon, they realized how much they had in common and how much they enjoyed each other's conversation. After Dave had come to visit Jenny several times, he invited her to a weekend at his place, and she accepted. When he picked her up at the airport, she was happy to see him and looking forward to the weekend.

When they arrived at Dave's house, Jenny wasn't so sure. Dave's house was such a cluttered mess, she could barely make her way to the guest room. There were piles of papers tumbling over almost every surface—from the coffee table in the living room to the kitchen table to the bathroom counter. There were two piles of laundry on the couch. And boxes piled up by the back door. Jenny's apartment was by no means spotless, but she had never seen a mess as big as this. It really made her uncomfortable.

"Yeah, the place is kind of a mess. Sorry about that," Dave said when he noticed the look on Jenny's face. "I really meant to clean it up for you, but I got so busy at work, I just didn't have time. I keep trying to get to the bottom of these piles of papers, but I just can't seem to get rid of them."

Jenny didn't know what to say.

Although people with ADD don't necessarily like living with so much clutter, they often have such great difficulty organizing their lives that they just can't seem to get out from under it all. It's not uncommon for them to have stacks and stacks of old magazines, laundry piled everywhere, bills piled everywhere, and boxes and boxes of "stuff" in the attic and the basement. It is a situation that just seems to get worse and worse, and never really resolved. It's easy to get overwhelmed and even walk away from the situation when it seems so impossible to fix.

In terms of ADD, what is happening to Dave is a combination of a couple of different ADD traits. Difficulty with organization—it's conception and execution. And then there are other distractions like the doorbell ringing, the phone ringing, the anxiety he feels as he realizes there are some very important papers he needs . . . and those papers are still at his office. Put them together and what does that spell? Clutter, anxiety, and disaster . . . especially for someone like Jenny, who really can't stand to be around that kind of clutter.

6) "I love her, but she's the most disorganized person I've ever met in my life." (Disorganization.)

Lonnie figures that he had been in love with Roberta for twenty-five years before he got her to marry him. He fell in love with her in grade school, when they were both ten years old. And he knew then that he wanted to be with her every moment of his life. But she wasn't as interested in Lonnie, and they each went on to marry other people. At age thirty, they were both divorced and happened to run into each other at the grocery store. Within a few months, they were dating, and Lonnie had never been happier. After all, Roberta had always been the girl of his dreams. He had never stopped thinking of her. And she was even more wonderful than he had remembered.

One of the things that Lonnie loved about Roberta was her sense of adventure and her spontaneity. At the proverbial drop of a hat, she would suggest that they drive out of town for the weekend. She teased Lonnie that he had never learned how to really enjoy life because he had always been planning it to death.

"Relax," she told him. "Open up. So what if we don't have a confirmation number for the hotel reservations. Let's just get in the car and go. We can worry about the rest of it later." She called it "Zen traveling."

Lonnie did loosen up a lot and found that he was having more fun than he could have imagined. It was a new experience for him to just trust Roberta and not worry about the organizational details that he usually spent so much time on.

Things were great between them for several years—until they got married. On the two-month anniversary of their marriage, the electricity went off in their house. Roberta, who had said she would take care of paying the bills the previous month, had misplaced the electricity bill and it had never been paid. Lonnie was stunned.

"How could you just forget to pay a bill?" he asked her. "Where is it? Give it to me and I'll go down there and pay it right now."

"I'm sorry. I just got busy with work. It's not such a big deal," she said. But then she couldn't find the bill when she went to look for it. She couldn't find her car keys, either. And when Lonnie walked outside to cool off for a minute, he couldn't believe what he saw.

"Roberta, what the heck is this?" he asked. "Could you come out here and explain this to me?"

"What are you talking about?" she asked as she came outside.

Lonnie pointed to a large watermelon sitting in the middle of their driveway. Roberta immediately went over to it. "Oh, there it is!" she said. "I wondered what had happened to that. I knew I bought a watermelon this afternoon. But when I got in the house I couldn't find it with the other groceries. I must have put it there when I was unloading the car." Lonnie just stared at her.

Many people with ADD are extremely disorganized because they don't pay close attention (as in attention deficit disorder) to what they're doing at the moment. Chances are that by the time Roberta got around to unloading the groceries, her mind was on twenty other things. Her hands were full, and she probably stuck the watermelon in the first place she could find while she fumbled for her keys, her purse, and another bag of groceries. She may have had mail in her hand at the time (she's not certain whether she did or not), and she has no idea where she put that down—including, of course, the bills that came that day. To her amazement, when she put the watermelon in the refrigerator, she found not only the mail, but her car keys too.

People with ADD very commonly misplace their keys, their mail, their wallets, checkbooks, gloves, hats, hairbrush, bills, cards, etc. Anything that is easy to pick up and put down in a new place, and that isn't heavy enough to require much thought, is likely to get misplaced. And the result is the tremendous frustration and exhaustion that comes from never being able to find what you need when you need it—or from living with someone whose life seems to be always on the verge of organizational collapse.

7) "But you said you loved me." (Difficulty staying on task— including staying on task in relationships.)

When Denny and Suzanne began dating, Suzanne thought she was probably the happiest and luckiest woman on the face of the planet. Denny was the kindest, most attentive and romantic man she had ever met. He deluged her with flowers, love notes, romantic weekend getaways. He cooked for her, cleaned for her, and spent time with her every chance he could get. He said he could never get enough of her. And she felt the same way about him.

Five months after they met, Denny asked Suzanne to marry him. She said yes, although she realized she hadn't known him that long. But she couldn't imagine not spending the rest of her life with this wonderful, caring, and romantic man. So they set the date for the wedding, reserved the church, hired a photographer, ordered the invitations, the cake . . . and then everything suddenly changed.

Denny wasn't calling as often as he had. He didn't come by to see her constantly as he had before. He was too busy to get together, or he had to work, he said. Suzanne was both hurt and worried. But when she asked Denny about these behaviors, he told her he loved her just as much as ever. Suzanne had no idea what to do. What had happened to the wonderfully romantic and caring Denny she thought she knew and loved? And in light of this recent change in behavior, what would life be like if they went ahead with the wedding and got married?

Denny probably did care about Suzanne just as much as he did before. But Denny was getting bored. And his boredom had nothing to do with Suzanne. It had to do with his ADD and the constant need for stimulation. This might be the saddest of all problems in ADD relationships. Just about the time the relationship begins to grow to a deeper level, the ADD partner may become bored and mistake their boredom for a loss of love—because they've "lost that lovin' feeling." Often, when the feelings leave, so does the ADD partner.

Denny was genuinely attracted to Suzanne when they first met and were first dating, and he felt a tremendous love for her. But, without realizing it, Denny was drawn to the *stimulation* of those feelings just as much as he was drawn to Suzanne.

When we fall in love, our bodies produce biochemicals called endorphins. These are biochemical agents that make us feel warm and fuzzy all over. Everyone—whether they have ADD or not—will most likely experience these "love feelings" generated by biochemistry. But people with ADD are often more attracted to those love feelings because of the stimulating effect on their brain.

Denny loved the endorphin rush he got from that wonderful feeling of new love. In fact, he was self-medicating his ADD with endorphins. But when the newness of the situation wore off a bit, the relationship wasn't as exciting for him as it had been initially. When Denny became what he thought was bored, in reality he was experiencing a lack of neurobiological stimulation.

The endorphin rush wasn't there for him anymore, and that scared Denny as much as his change in behavior scared Suzanne. Denny began to get cold feet because there were no biochemical reactions taking place in his body—the endorphin rush—to help him feel "normal." For a lot of ADD folks, because we are predominantly kinesthetic learners, the way we experience reality is through visceral feelings, more so than the linear logic of commitment.

A kinesthetic learner is someone who learns through "body understandings." Linear learners understand life through their linear thought processes. Whereas a linear learner can hear the statement, "Don't touch the stove because it is hot," and understand it without having to touch the stove, that same statement would make no sense whatsoever to the kinesthetic learner unless they touch the stove. They need that "body experience" to comprehend what the linear learner understood simply through linear logic: stove + hot = burn. In reality, we may have traits of both learning styles, but usually people are more linear than kinesthetic, or vice versa.

In this case, Denny's understanding of love was directly tied to his feelings—his body understanding. So when the feelings were gone, the logical assumption was that the love was gone. Linear learners would also feel the endorphin rush, but when the intense feelings die down, their linear logic would take over and tell them that love was more than just a feeling.

Modern-day psychotherapy encourages people to be in touch with their feelings and then follow their feelings. Unfortunately, someone with ADD may have the roughest experience imaginable. When based on endorphins, their feelings can take them around corners with twists and turns you'd never believe were possible. Denny was trying to be in touch with his feelings. But his feelings were scaring the bejeebers out of him. Why? He understands his world through his feelings (kinesthetic learning). And when his feelings are tied directly to endorphins experienced or not experienced in the relationship, this can terrify both partners.

The lack of endorphins rushing through Denny's body was a marker for him that indicated he was jumping into this relationship too fast and had made a wrong decision in choosing Suzanne to be his bride. Since the thrill was gone, that had to mean that the love was gone too. Although this was not the case, for Denny it sure felt like it.

Suzanne was the same person she had been four months earlier. And Denny's genuine attraction to Suzanne was still there. But his attraction to the stimulation of the relationship was gone. And his boredom—his lack of stimulation—made him feel trapped. He didn't know what to do. Should he follow through with his plans to marry Suzanne? She was a wonderful lady. But Denny was bored. And he needed a new source of stimulation. He needed to find that next rush—that next fix, if you wish. Only that isn't what Denny thought he was really after. He thought he was seeking a genuine, mutually satisfying relationship with someone he wanted to spend the rest of his life with.

Genuinely caring. Wonderful. Romantic. Thoughtful. Scared. Denny was all of the above . . . and very ADD.

8) "If I say black, she says white." (Argumentative. Conflict-seeking.)

Roger absolutely could not understand what was happening in his marriage. He knew he loved Nancy and he knew she loved him. But they seemed to have a pattern of incessant arguing that he just didn't know how to break. He didn't want to argue with her about every little thing. He knew it wasn't good for the kids, and it didn't feel good to him, either. But no matter what he said to Nancy, she found some way to argue with him about it. And it didn't matter what the subject was. She would argue about work, about meals, about the house, the kids, the dog—even the weather.

"Look at what a beautiful day it is," Roger would say.

"How can you say it's beautiful with this breeze blowing around?" she'd answer.

"It's just a breeze, not a wind storm," he'd say.

"You can call it what you want, but it's certainly not beautiful. This is just not beautiful weather. I can't stand it. It's sunny day after day. We need some rain."

"But you don't like it when it's raining. You say you can't stand stormy weather."

"No I don't. I never complain about the rain."

And Roger would give up. Sometimes he would be exhausted from arguing before any of them even left the house in the morning for work or school. And he just couldn't understand what was happening.

Nancy argued constantly for the same reason that Denny initially threw himself so completely into his relationship with Suzanne. It all comes back to that need for stimulation. Remember this next statement—it will help you understand a lot of what goes on for people with ADD: "Stimulation is my friend." Although people with ADD don't usually realize it, they will seek stimulation in any way possible. It doesn't matter if it is positive stimulation or negative stimulation. To some degree, stimulation is stimulation. Conflict-seeking—arguing—is one of many ways to be stimulated. The confrontation puts them into a fight-or-flight modality. Adrenaline, a neurostimulant, is released into the bloodstream and instantly, there is the stimulation they need. When their brain is stimulated, they feel better in their body.

"Feeling better in their body" is an extremely important concept in understanding what the ADD person experiences. This is not a "touchy-feely" concept here. We are talking about feelings that have both a psychological and a concrete physical component to them.

For example, when you have the flu, you experience physical discomfort because there is a physical problem: the flu. The same is true for people with ADD. In addition to the behaviors and emotions caused by ADD, the disorder also has a component of physical discomfort. But this is a physical discomfort they are often never even aware of, because they were born with ADD and have no other experience in their body to compare it with.

If you are not ADD and you have never had that feeling, I wish I could describe it to you. But I really can't. It's not an achy feeling, or an itchy feeling. It isn't a feeling of pain or hunger or arousal. But it is a very real physical feeling of discomfort. And we refer to it as a feeling of "discomfort in the person's body." Conversely, when someone with ADD is diagnosed and treated with medication, they often begin to feel "comfortable in their body" for the first time in their life.

When people with ADD engage in activities to provide stimulation for their brain, even activities like arguing, they usually do feel better in their bodies. The problem, of course, is that their partner, their children, or anyone on the receiving end of conflict-seeking behavior usually doesn't feel better. If anything, they feel frustrated, exhausted, and a whole lot worse. After enough arguing with their partner, exhausted and stressed out from the constant conflict, they might not be sure the relationship is even worth it. That doesn't sound like a whole lot of fun for anyone. Nancy would much prefer to have positive stimulation. But, stimulation is stimulation no matter how you get it.

So Nancy self-medicates, through conflict-seeking behaviors which release adrenaline into her system, and then she gets to feel better in her body. But Nancy has problems with two parts of her brain. She has decreased activity in her prefrontal cortex and increased activity in her cingulate gyrus. As we discussed earlier in this chapter, this pattern is referred to as the overfocused subtype of ADD. Nancy's prefrontal cortex is the stimulation-seeking element in her behaviors, and her cingulate keeps her stuck in the whole process. So once she takes a stance in an argument, she gets stuck in her thinking and can't shift from that stance. Even when she would like to shift, she just keeps arguing and can't let go.

When the individual who has ADD also has this extra oomph— or drive, if you wish—from the cingulate, it makes things worse in many ways. On the other hand, Nancy is an accountant and needs to be very exacting in her work. She needs her cingulate to give her the stick-to-it-iveness required to track every red cent that has been spent and know exactly how and why it was spent. Her overactive cingulate makes her a consummate professional in the accounting world. She knows which pigeonhole to pigeonhole entries into so everything balances. She reads over contracts for her clients with a fine-toothed comb—often catching things their attorney didn't catch. She's very good at her profession because of her overactive cingulate. Unfortunately, this is that very same brain system that also causes her to be argumentative and anything but successful in her personal and family life.

9) "He's got a one-track mind." (Hyperfocused.)

Heather and Martin had been married for about two years when Martin decided he wanted to learn to sail. Although Heather wasn't really interested in it herself, she enjoyed it vicariously through Martin. He bought books, took lessons, and seemed to thrive on his newfound love of sailing. Wishing to be supportive, Heather often went sailing with Martin.

Several months after he started taking lessons, Martin announced that he wanted them to buy their own sailboat. For weeks, that was about all he could talk about. Heather wasn't sure how they were going to afford to buy the boat, but this seemed to make Martin happy and excited, so she tried to go along with it. She tried to be supportive and encouraging, and she listened to his constant talk about sailing and sailboats. When she would suggest they go to a movie, he suggested going down to the marina instead. When she asked him to go with her to an office party, he said he would love to go, but he had an appointment with a broker to look at a used boat that was a really good deal.

Just when Heather began to feel that she couldn't stand one more minute of his talk about sailing, Martin stopped talking about sailing. All of sudden, he wasn't interested in sailing anymore. He stopped talking about buying a boat. He stopped going down to the marina. He didn't go sailing on weekends.

Instead, Martin started to play roller hockey. A friend of his took him to a roller hockey game, and Martin immediately fell in love with the sport. He bought hundreds of dollars worth of skates and equipment, joined the league, and started practicing three nights a week. On weekends, he would hang out at the rink, watching other teams play before his own game. On weeknights, he would watch ice hockey on TV. He bought books about hockey and studied catalogs of hockey equipment for hours at a time.

Heather was just as confused as she had been during Martin's sailing days. Why did he always have to become so totally involved and immersed in any one activity? What was the matter with him? "What's the matter with me?" she thought. "What's wrong with me that he doesn't focus on me once in a while?"

Martin's hyperfocused behavior is very common for someone with ADD. People with ADD can become hyperfocused on hobbies, work, the family next door—just as they were hyperfocused on their mate at the beginning of the relationship. The main issue, here again, is the need for stimulation. And when they become so familiar with a person or an activity that it no longer provides that stimulation, they move on to the next stimulating event.

When we looked at Nancy, the woman who always sought conflict, we saw "overfocused" behaviors. In this story we read about "hyperfocus." What's the difference between these two?

Hyperfocus comes from that physical need for stimulation. The behaviors associated with hyperfocus serve only to increase activity in the prefrontal cortex—where ADD originates. Those are the kinds of behaviors we saw in Martin, who hyperfocused in one area as long as it was stimulating. Once the stimulation is gone (once the activity has lost its excitement), so is Martin. Overfocus, on the other hand, comes from the person's inability to shift focus. A person who is overfocused gets locked-in on something and stays that way—not primarily because they need the stimulation, but because they just can't shift gears in their mind. Their brain won't let them.

If you're thinking that the distinction between hyperfocus and overfocus is difficult to grasp, you're right. It is difficult to identify and understand the subtle but significant difference between these two types of behavior. And that is yet another reason it is important to have a trained professional diagnosing and treating ADD.

Both hyperfocus and overfocus can be working together at the same time. When that happens, the person may hyperfocus to experience stimulation, but then end up overfocusing on it because they can't shift away from it. It's a double whammy. Sorry, no one said you only get one problem with the metabolic uptake in your brain. One or more brain systems can be involved with ADD. But take heart. There is hope. We'll talk about some of that hope towards the end of this chapter.

10) "She's just so incredibly inconsiderate." (All the above traits combined into one person.)

So what happens when you put all these ADD traits together in a mate? You often get someone who doesn't follow through with commitments, gets bored with their mate, gets stuck in their thinking, and is disorganized, forgetful, routinely late, and argumentative. In other words, you have someone who might be a wonderful person, but whose outward behaviors look inconsiderate—day after day after day. It's not a pretty picture. And it's certainly not easy to live with. Come to think of it, this sounds a lot like the Wilsons we met in Chapter One.

So Now What Should I Do?

Now that you've read through this checklist of ADD behaviors, you might be thinking that you and every single person you know has ADD. After all, which of us hasn't lost our car keys from time to time or longed for the physical rush of new love? Which of us hasn't argued with our mate, forgotten appointments, or forgotten to pay a bill?

The truth is that all of us have some of these traits from time to time. But if you or your mate has a lot of these traits a lot of the time, then one of you probably needs to be professionally evaluated for ADD.

The bad news is that these ADD traits can make relationships a living hell. The good news is that ADD is a medical condition, not a character flaw. As a medical condition, most often it can be treated with medication. And when ADD is treated, many of these difficult traits can either diminish or be eliminated.

If your partner has ADD, it really comes down to these two questions for you: 1) If you really love this person, are you able to be clear about the fact that these ADD problems are problems of the brain, not of the heart? and 2) If this person were to never change, could you spend the rest of your life with them, accepting them for who they are—ADD and all?

Of course, there are no right or wrong answers to either of these questions. But if you do have an ADD partner, then these are important questions you really need to ask yourself . . . and answer for yourself.

If you are the ADD person, there are also a couple of questions you need to ask yourself: 1) Knowing that you are driving other people to extremes with your ADD behaviors—often hurting them, though unintentionally—do you really want to keep doing that? and 2) What are you willing to do to change? See a doctor? Take medication? Learn communication skills? Change can be scary. Admitting you have a problem can be scary. But what is worse? Admitting that you have a problem or continuing to be a problem? I encourage you to opt for the "I have a problem" category. It puts you into a greater position of power to overcome the problem.

"I have a problem called ADD. My ADD is not me, but it is a part of me. I didn't choose to have ADD. It came from my parent's gene pool. That doesn't make me a problem. It makes me a person with a problem." When we look at it that way, the only real challenge is doing something about the problem. And that is usually an easier problem to solve. Maybe this will make more sense if you first know a little more about ADD in general.

You've read through the previous checklist and feel that it describes you or your mate in many ways. And you think maybe you or they might have ADD. But using the checklist above is not the way to diagnose ADD. Hopefully it has heightened your awareness of ADD-like symptoms, but just because you can relate to many (if not every) of the characteristics above doesn't give you a diagnosis of ADD. In order for there to be an actual diagnosis, you need to be evaluated by a clinician who can make such a diagnosis: a physician (M.D.), a psychiatrist (M.D.), a psychologist (Ph.D.), a licensed marriage and family counselor (L.M.F.C.C.), or a licensed clinical social worker (L.C.S.W.). These are the professionals who have the credentials to diagnose. But even then, their credentials are often not enough to go by because of a lag in the information curve many clinicians have. Just having the license is not enough. You really need to see someone who specializes in evaluating ADD. You want someone who has spent lots of time studying on their own about ADD—going to conferences and professional training seminars about ADD. You want someone who has a large number of ADD patients in their practice, someone who has tons of experience evaluating and treating ADD. You need someone with significant ADD experience because the traits of ADD are often subtle and can vary greatly from person to person. To complicate matters even more, the expression of those traits can even vary significantly from time to time within one individual. If these prerequisites are not met among the physicians in your area, then see if you can find a doctor who doesn't know it all and is willing to immerse himself (or herself), for your sake, in educating himself about ADD. The current research. The current interventions. The nuances of ADD that the average clinician doesn't notice unless he has such an education.

There is no comprehensive and definitive "test" used to evaluate and diagnose ADD. The diagnosis of ADD is based on the individual's behavioral history. Clinicians have set diagnostic criteria from which a diagnosis of ADD can or can't be made. It is standardized diagnostic criteria used universally throughout the clinical community. The symptoms of ADD must have been present (in one form or another) since the age of seven. ADD is not something you mysteriously develop when you are thirty-five. It just doesn't work that way, unless there has been some sort of head trauma. And even then, even if the symptoms are the same, head trauma is likely to be given a different diagnostic label. Most likely, either you were born with it, or you don't have it. Or you may have a mild version of ADD which can make it much more difficult to diagnose. Or you've compensated for it your whole life and only now realize you have ADD.

The good news is that because ADD is a medical condition, it can be treated medically. Since the causes of ADD behaviors are an inadequate supply of the neurotransmitter dopamine in the brain and decreased activity in the prefrontal cortex, we can begin to solve the problem by increasing the amount of dopamine. Get the phone lines back up and working, so to speak, so the prefrontal cortex can process information and the individual can function better.

There are basically five medications used as a first-line defense to treat classic ADD. They are Ritalin (methylphenidate), Dexedrine (dextroamphetamine), Adderall (amphetamine salts), Cylert (pemoline), and Desoxyn (methamphetamine). All of these medications have been thoroughly tested and re-tested to make certain that the medications do what they are supposed to do. They have been researched extensively under strict ruling from the Federal Drug Administration (FDA) to ensure that they are safe for the American public. The chances of any of these medications having any serious lifelong effect are slim to none when taken as prescribed at a therapeutic dose for that patient's brain. Which medication is best? If you have ADD, it's the one that works best for you. What dose should you take? The one prescribed by your physician. You have hired the services of a physician to treat you medically for your ADD. If you have followed the ideas above in terms of finding a competent doctor to treat your ADD, you should be in good hands. Everybody's body is different. You might do well on Adderall and your friend who also has ADD might do better on Ritalin. It just depends upon your body and your brain.

Now then: There are other medications which can be used to treat ADD, but they are more of a second-line defense. These medications may be prescribed instead of the first five listed above when the physician is concerned that a neurostimulant would be contraindicated. What should you take? Again, that's between you and your physician. Some of these second-line defenses include (but are not limited to) Effexor (venlafaxine) and Wellbutrin (bupropion hydrochloride), which are two very specific types of antidepressants. And then there are medications to help tone down hyperactive ADD behaviors, like Catapres (clonidine) and Tenex (guanfacine), which are actually high blood pressure medications. There are even trials of Aricept (donepezil hydrochloride) being used to some success in treating ADD. Aricept is actually a medication used to treat Alzheimer's patients. So if your physician is choosing to use second-line defense medications to treat your ADD, you of course would want to ask him why. But you also need to realize that some medications used for other specific medical conditions are sometimes used for treating ADD. What should you take? That's a medical question—one that is better answered by your physician than in a book such as this.

Just because you have decreased activity in your prefrontal cortex—ADD—doesn't mean you can't have some other problem co-existing in another part (or parts) of your brain at the same time. Often, people who have ADD do have problems with other brain systems besides their prefrontal cortex. Remember Nancy? That was the case with her brain. Decreased activity of the prefrontal cortex (ADD) and increased activity of her cingulate (overfocused).

Sometimes doctors need to prescribe more than one type of medication to help people function better in life. Using Nancy, for example, who has problems with both her prefrontal cortex and her cingulate, the physician might need to prescribe both a neurostimulant and a special kind of antidepressant—an SSRI—that will simultaneously decrease the overactivity of her cingulate. SSRI is medical shorthand for Serotonin Selective Reuptake Inhibitor. Brand name medications that are SSRIs are medications like Prozac, Zoloft, and Luvox. These medications can often make the overfocused behaviors—the argumentativeness, worry, "stuck in their thinking" behaviors—diminish if not go away completely. That could be a wonderful change for Nancy and her family.

There are other brain systems which may not be working as they are supposed to and may also require some sort of medication as an intervention to make things better. I am telling you all of this because I want you and/or your significant other to be prepared for other possible strategies your physician may want to prescribe in treating the ADD. If you are the one who has ADD, a competent physician can work with you to determine the most effective regimen of medication or medications needed for you. You've probably got a great brain, but it just needs some fine tuning.

Take a deep breath. Relax. Chances are you'll be just fine when in the hands of a competent physician who knows ADD inside and out and knows the best protocols for treating not just ADD, but your specific kind of ADD.

Medication is the solution of choice for addressing the problems associated with ADD. However, many people with ADD are not on the appropriate medication. Some have not yet been properly diagnosed, others are being seen by doctors or therapists who might not have the most up-to-date information on the medical treatment of ADD, and some people might be "against" taking medication for personal reasons. Although they might not be on medication, many of these people are still trying to increase their dopamine level—although they might not even realize it.

Some people increase their dopamine level by seeking stimulation. Usually that means increasing the body's output of adrenaline, and adrenaline can be used as a neurostimulant to increase activity in the brain.

Remember Nancy, the woman who argued over everything, including the weather? Nancy's conflict-seeking behaviors were very stimulating. She went into fight-or-flight mode, raised her adrenaline level, and used adrenaline to increase the activity in her brain. She didn't realize consciously what she was doing. But she kept repeating her behaviors on a subconscious level because she recognized that in some way it made her feel better. In fact, one time in an argument with her husband (who was exhausted from all the arguing), Nancy stated: "I like to argue. I feel good when I argue!" Bottom line, she just wanted to feel better in her body. There's certainly no fault in that. Unfortunately, it was causing major turmoil in her romantic relationship with Roger.

Research supports the concept of self-medicating with adrenaline. Years ago a study was done in which the urine of non-ADD children and the urine of ADD children was tested and compared to see if there were any significant differences between the two groups. There was only one significant difference: the ADD children had a higher level of adrenaline in their urine—adrenaline that was produced in their bodies through their hyperactive/impulsive behaviors and used to self-medicate their prefrontal cortex.

Other ways that people self-medicate is through the use of drugs like nicotine and caffeine. Nicotine and caffeine are easily accessible and both are neurostimulants. But they are not very good neurostimulants, as neurostimulants go, in that the individual experiences highs and lows as long as the caffeine or nicotine is present in their body. They're not consistent in their overall effect. Plus, we already know that nicotine and caffeine are not the best substances to put into one's body. There is a long list of deadly diseases associated with nicotine. Caffeine also has major negative effects in the body over a lifetime of abuse. But . . . if it's all you've got available to you, and you need to get your brain running better so you can feel better in your body and perform better . . . you're likely to use whatever you can get your hands on.

And that's another reason that medical treatment—for this medical condition—is so important.

THREE

Avoid Making Poor Partnering Decisions

I know a woman who is now in her fourth marriage. And she still has no idea how she ended up choosing the wrong mate at least three times. Hopefully, the fourth time's the charm.

Tina, forty-five, married her first husband straight out of high school. They had been sweethearts since the ninth grade. On a whim, they ran off and got married on graduation night after all the festivities were over. They were very much in love, she says, but his mother made their lives miserable, and they divorced the following year.

Next, Tina married a guy she met at the hardware store. She had gone in to buy some floor tiles and started flirting with the salesman. They started dating and were married six months later. That marriage lasted for three years. For two of those years, her husband was abusive. Tina says now that she doesn't know why she married him and doesn't know why she stayed with him. But she did.

At that point, Tina decided to stay single. But when she turned thirty-five, she started to worry that she would never get married or have children. She met a cute guy on her company's softball team and married him the following year. He had two grown children from a previous marriage. Tina found out the year after they were married he was definitely not interested in any more children. Tina stayed with him for ten years, although she says she was miserable for nine of them. Then she got divorced.

This time, Tina decided to head for church. She dated several men she met at church and ended up marrying one of them. A few months after they married, he lost his job and has been working odd jobs in and out of town since then. Tina says she's happy, but she wishes her new husband was in town more often.

When I talk to her, she still doesn't know why she made so many poor choices over a period of almost thirty years.

Tina isn't all that different from the rest of us. True, most of us don't get divorced three times. But many of us do wake up at some point and wonder why we married the person we married in the first place. Why did we choose *this* person and promise to spend the rest of our lives with them? How did it happen?

People with ADD are even more likely than the general population to wake up one day with that question. Let's take a look at why.

1) The need for constant stimulation.

I've said it before and I'll say it again: Stimulation is my friend. People with ADD want, crave, need, and absolutely have to have stimulation. They are drawn to new stimulation like the proverbial moth to the flame. In many situations, of course, there is absolutely nothing wrong with needing and being attracted to stimulation. The problem for people with ADD is that the experience of new stimulation often blinds them to quite a few other aspects of their situation.

Because of this craving for stimulation, an ADD person will choose a partner who 1) is stimulating for them, 2) can "co-stimulate" with them, or 3) is willing to put up with their constant need for stimulation—someone who also seeks stimulation (perhaps a mate who also has ADD) and will partner with them in creating/seeking stimulation.

If their partner is stimulating for them, then the ADD person will use their partner to self-medicate their brain with endorphins and adrenaline and all the other good stuff that goes along with courting and romance. People with ADD seriously get into the stimulation of courting. In fact, you have never truly been courted and romanced until you have been courted and romanced by someone with ADD—someone who is hyperfocused on romancing you. This is the stuff Hollywood movies are made of. We're talking flowers and phone calls and picnics on the beach and poetry and billboards with messages of "I love you" and even sky-writing. When someone with ADD is romancing you in the courting process, birds whistle a happier melody, angels sing, and air smells sweeter. Every day is a special day because you are both so much in love. When hyperfocused on romance, men and women with ADD do the most fabulous, sweet, loving, nurturing things—because it is stimulating.

Yes, they do it because it is stimulating for *them*. They don't do it just because their partner will enjoy it, although that certainly is part of the reason they do it. But the biggest reason they sweep you off your feet with this incredible display of affection is because they are doing it for themselves, to self-medicate their brains with endorphins. They aren't trying to be selfish or self-centered. But they do all this courting and romancing to the hilt because it feels good for them to be stimulated by the excitement of romance. Mind you, this "it feels good" aspect is not just about your average "it makes me feel good to do something nice for the one I love." Also included in this mix is "I feel better in my own body"—a general, overall sense of well-being the person with ADD may not experience on a day-to-day basis like most of the population. That's a huge part of the attraction to self-medicating with romance. The individual gets to feel better in their own body—an experience they don't often achieve because their brain isn't working right. It's hard to feel good in your body when your brain doesn't work the way it's supposed to.

The person on the receiving end of this courting process doesn't realize that most of this attention has less to do with them than they think. In fact, they usually think it's all about them. And why wouldn't they?

But the ADD person wouldn't be able to tell you it's about self-medicating either. They are clueless as to why they're so enthralled with their newfound love. All they know is that the feelings they are having are so intense, so wonderful, that this person has to be their soulmate. The one perfect person God has specifically chosen for them. They are in no way conscious of the self-medicating aspect of what they are doing. After all, they're in love. And love is about giving, about intense feelings and keeping the fire of their romance stoked and in full blaze. There is no way that they would consciously, knowingly, do all of these things just to use their partner to self-medicate. That would be using someone for personal gain. The average ADD person wouldn't stand for that because it is altruistically wrong. But . . .

The problem is that the feelings they have—the rush of endorphins—are so strong. People with ADD tend to be kinesthetic learners. They understand life better when it is interpreted through their body experiences. So naturally, these fabulous feelings are interpreted as true love. They have strong feelings of "love" for the person they are romancing, and the more they romance them the stronger the feelings get. And the more they romance them, the more their partner responds in a similar fashion. It's a mutually satisfying relationship, and both want that experience to go on for the rest of their lives together.

Unfortunately, the ADD partner goes on and on with all this exciting courtship stuff until it becomes a commonplace experience. And when it loses its newness—when it is no longer stimulating   it simply stops. Sometimes immediately. One day they're full of love, birds and angels singing and all, and the next day, nothing. Gone. Zilch. Zero.

When the thrill is gone, the thrill is gone. The ADD partner no longer writes the poetry or the songs or sends romantic phone messages because they aren't getting the rush anymore. And when it isn't stimulating to them anymore, they simply stop those behaviors and move on to something else. They may, in fact, be very much in love with their partner, but the stimulation is gone. In order to feel better—okay in their own body—they've got to find something else that is stimulating. It's also possible that once the feelings are gone, they believe the love is also gone. They become terrified of yet another disastrous relationship (it's usually happened several times before) and leave post haste, before any further serious damage occurs.

Of course the object of all the previous attention and affection is usually stunned at this point. Up to this point, their mate has been more than they had ever dreamed of. Then, suddenly, he or she just isn't there anymore. The non-ADD partner ends up sitting in the dust of an illusion asking themselves what went wrong. They are confused. They are hurt. They are bewildered. And they are angry.

Amazingly, the ADD partner is also feeling confused by this time, too. Here they thought they had found the mate of their dreams. This was the most stimulating relationship they had ever been in. Then, suddenly, those feelings were gone. If they were married during this intense courtship phase—which often happens—then both partners could be panicking at this point.

Of course, all the romancing and courting behavior just might have been reflective of the ADD partner's true feelings. Maybe this really was the right mate for them. Maybe they really do want the relationship to work. Certainly they had no idea that they were lavishing all this attention on their mate only because it felt good for them to do so—that all these feelings were just an attempt to med-icate a metabolic deficiency on their part.

Nevertheless, you can easily see how a relationship could be in some serious trouble by this time.

The second aspect of how ADD influences the choice of a mate happens when people with ADD are looking for a partner they can be stimulating with, not just someone they can lavish attention on. A sort of co-creating of stimulation.

For example, prior to my marriage to Terri, one woman I dated told me she had more "lifetime experiences" with me in the first six months of our relationship than she had with her former husband in their ten years of marriage. We went places. Did things. Had fun. Went out. Stayed in. Traveled all over. Why? I craved the stimula-tion. I had an incredible resume of life experiences (a sometimes beneficial aspect of ADD) based on stimulation-seeking behaviors. Plus, I think she had a few stimulation-seeking urges as well.

In this kind of relationship, if one partner asks, "Hey, you want to go to Disneyland this weekend?" there's no partner there to say, "Are you nuts? Do you realize how far behind both of us are in our bills already?" Instead, both partners co-create stimulation. They both use the relationship to create the stimulation they need to feel better in their own bodies. They both enjoy themselves. They both add to the stimulation by charging even more on their already over-taxed credit cards (that'll get the adrenaline going the day the bills arrive). And they both use each other to do all of this without real-izing why.

This can be a very fun-loving, exciting relationship that can last a lifetime when there really is mutual love and respect for each other. Never a dull moment, as the saying goes. It's important to realize (as we'll see more clearly in Chapter Seven) that not all of this stimulation-seeking behavior is bad. A lot of it can add won-derful dimensions to a relationship and help make it last a lifetime. Mutually satisfying co-created stimulation can be one of those positive attributes. But it can just as easily take away from the satisfaction if things like spending impulsively are not kept in check. Whereas years ago the most common reason for irreconcilable differences was sex, nowadays it is most often about money.

The third area in which stimulation is involved in the selection of a mate occurs when the ADD partner is drawn to someone who can tolerate their constant need for stimulation. In this case, the non-ADD partner usually provides some type of structure for the relationship within which the ADD partner can have the spontaneity and stimulation they want and need. They become the anchor of stability, so to speak, that allows the ADD person to soar to their highest potential without getting so far out there that they lose their way. They become the safety net to catch their ADD partner should they start to fall.

This may sound a bit codependent, but in this specific example, it is more about the non-ADD partner enjoying experiences in life they have never known, experiences the ADD partner brings to the relationship that enhance the relationship and their lives together as a couple.

A non-ADD partner who is willing to put up with his partner's constant need for stimulation really needs to have a good solid base in reality and know when and how to help steer things away to calmer waters from time to time. When this method of choosing a partner—someone who can put up with the stimulation—is sealed with real friendship and facilitated as a partnership, it can be one of the richest, most fulfilling kinds of relationships there is.

On the other hand, if the ADD and non-ADD partner are not in a working partnership in which both people know their roles, the non-ADD partner may get tired of always having to reel in their ADD partner. They may become frustrated with the impulsiveness and craziness that can erupt with this kind of combination. They end up feeling as if they have to control their ADD partner and hate that role.

Likewise, the ADD person may feel controlled and stifled. They may panic at the loss of approval to be spontaneous—and be spontaneous, they must. They feel as if they're with a schoolteacher and they are the student. Unless they are able to form a synergistic partnership in which they both take advantage of each other's strengths and weaknesses, the relationship is likely to be much less than satisfying and eventually blow apart.

2) The lack of impulse control.

Remember Tina, the woman who had been married four times? Her very first marriage—and possibly each of the other three, also—was a perfect example of a classic symptom of ADD, and one that gets people in trouble again and again. Poor impulse control. There she was on graduation night with her boyfriend of four years at an all-night graduation party. Out of nowhere, he suggests to Tina that they get married that very night.

"Fine," Tina says. "Do you really mean it?"

"Sure I do." They embrace passionately and kiss.

"Let's go for it right now," she says.

They get in the car and wake up the justice of the peace and two hours later, they're married. Talk about poor impulse control. Both Tina and her beau had the thought and immediately acted on it.

Another couple I know also got married on a whim because of lack of impulse control. This couple met for the very first time at a dance and got married *that very night*. These people knew each other for less than twenty-four hours when they made their vows to spend the rest of their lives together. After all, why wait? They felt such an attraction for each other. And that's such an intense and wonderful feeling. They wanted to keep that feeling for the rest of their lives. They were absolutely, totally sure of it. So why waste time getting to know each other, right? Their basic attitude was, "Hey, we like the feeling we have now. We want to keep it. Let's get married."

Now, really, how much sense does that make? Both of them (silently to themselves) had that same thought once the honeymoon phase was over.

This particular couple has been together now for twelve years. And they have two children. Their marriage isn't what I would call a satisfying relationship. But they are still together. That in itself is pretty amazing.

They literally lived out a fantasy from popular song lyrics. They spotted each other "across a crowded room." And that was it. They were completely convinced within minutes that this person was their soulmate, their one-and-only, their everything. Instant love. But it's not love based in reality. It is a mirage that disappears once the stimulation is gone and the partners have to start dealing with the realities of daily life with someone they barely know.

Of course, not everyone with ADD takes it quite that far. But lack of impulse control often does play a role when a person with ADD selects a mate. We see someone we're very attracted to, go out with them once, and then decide we are completely in love. Within weeks (possibly hours), we start to believe that this is the person we are going to marry. We fantasize about them and the bliss we will share the rest of our lives. And we often try to fool ourselves into believing that we actually do know what we're doing as we rush headlong into marriage. We tell ourselves that we have that special intuition that comes with ADD. And we buy into that and believe we can't possibly be making the wrong decision.

A lot of people with ADD do have a wonderful sense of intuition. That part of it is not fantasy. And our intuition might really be telling us that this person would be a good choice for our mate. Personally, I think that if you trust that intuition right away and it really does work out, you're lucky. Just because we have a wonderful sense of intuition doesn't mean it's always going to be accurate—especially if we're self-medicating with romance.

Getting married minutes after meeting someone really isn't a very common ADD behavior. It does happen, but it is not that common. But impulsivity does play a large role in the courting behavior I was discussing earlier. When you are endorphin-deprived, so to speak, and you find someone who is stimulating, your impulsivity increases your chances of jumping in head first. Remember: "Stimulation is my friend."

It's your impulsivity speaking when you call your girlfriend in the middle of the night and tell her to get ready because you're coming over to pick her up for a surprise trip to a quaint little romantic bed and breakfast. It's your impulsivity speaking when you see a sky-writer at the beach and immediately call the company to put your sweetheart's name up in the sky—no matter what it's going to cost. And it's your impulsivity speaking when you pass a flower vendor on the street and decide to buy an armload of roses and deliver them to your sweetheart at work right that very minute. Romantic? Yes, very. Stimulating? Absolutely. Love? Well, maybe. Time will tell.

Yes, all of those activities are stimulating. But if you had an appropriate amount of impulse control, you might consider whether or not they were wise moves before you jumped right into them. And if you had better impulse control, you might have made sure to get to know your mate better before you got married. You would have taken the time and made the effort that is required to really get to know someone. You might not have been so impatient and in such a hurry to skip right over the dating and go straight to the marriage. And that way, when the stimulation of the courting phase was over and the newness of the romance had worn off, you would be left with a person you knew well, liked, and respected— instead of a stranger you married on a whim one night after a dance.

3) Inattention to detail.

Because people with ADD tend to be hyperfocused in certain areas, they miss the details in other areas.

For example, suppose you're in your friend's brand-new car and going for a test drive. You're hyperfocused on the car itself. You notice the texture and smell of the leather. You examine the dash-board lights, try all the buttons, test out the air conditioner, set the radio channels, etc. You're so hyperfocused on the car itself, you might not notice that your friend just got his ear pierced. Under normal circumstances, if you had just seen your friend at a party or at work, you would definitely have noticed that earring. But here, in a new and stimulating environment, you are too hyperfocused to notice other details.

Inattention to detail is a very common issue faced by people with ADD. This is true if the ADD person is so hyperfocused (as in the example above) that he misses some details. But it is also true for the inattentive type of ADD where the person, in general, misses details—hyperfocused or not. Perhaps they're just too spaced-out to notice or attend to details.

Let's say you're out on a date. You're staring at each other throughout dinner—lots of conversation, lots of eye contact. But then you notice your boyfriend's eyes are looking elsewhere. You might notice it physically, but not pay much attention to it because your mind is elsewhere. Your mind is on him, the romance, how he looks, how you feel, the stimulation, etc. In reality, he might be staring at every other woman in the entire restaurant. But chances are, you're missing that information because of your lack of attention to detail. After you've been together for a while, however, you find out that your boyfriend—or husband by that time—is a huge flirt. And you can't stand it. But you didn't realize it earlier because of inattention to detail.

Maybe you're dating a woman and you never really picked up on the fact that every single time she's at a restaurant or a social function, she has a glass of wine in her hand. You certainly saw that with your eyes, but you didn't really notice it with your brain. After a while, after the newness of the relationship starts to fade, you realize she's always got a glass of wine in her had because she is an alcoholic. That's an important detail you may have missed until it was too late.

Whatever bothers you about your mate *after* marriage was probably present *before* you got married. You just didn't notice. It doesn't have to be anything as serious as alcoholism or inappropriate flirting. Maybe it's the laundry on the floor. The newspapers all over the kitchen counters. The weeds in the backyard. The dust on the lamp. The cap on (or off) the toothpaste tube.

If these are the kinds of things that will bother you in a marriage, you really need to be paying attention to these kinds of details during dating. But if you have ADD, that can be very difficult to do.

4) Unresolved conflicts with parents.

Many of us, in choosing a mate, are greatly influenced by conflicts with our parents that have remained unresolved. We might not recognize them as an influence in our lives. We might not even really want to think about it. But it's there, nevertheless. And while this issue is not unique to people who have ADD, it compounds their already difficult task of choosing a mate.

All of us have conflicts with our parents when we are children. Sometimes they're fairly superficial—we want to spend the night at Sally's but our mom won't let us. And sometimes they're much more serious—abuse, a divorce, or a death. But no matter what the conflict is, as children, we usually feel powerless to solve it. When we're children, we aren't able to stand up to our parents, to explain our needs clearly, and demand that our most important needs be met. We just know not to challenge our parents in that way. We need them in order for us to live—to survive. And so we don't stand up to them. But still, the feelings we have related to those life experiences are there, deep in our being. We have internalized those unresolved conflicts with the desire to someday find resolution. So when we grow up and search for a mate we can share the rest of our lives with, we subconsciously search for a partner who also embodies some of the same characteristics our parents did. We look for someone with some of the same positive and negative attributes of our parents. We gravitate to what's familiar to us when we're looking for a mate, no matter how functional or dysfunctional that person might be.

Partly what we are looking for is someone who has the same things "wrong" that our parents had "wrong." That way, we'll finally be able to resolve those issues and fix those things. That's because we'll be at a *peer level* with this person this time, instead of in the parent-child relationship where the parent has all the power and the child has none. The playing field will be even this time. This time, we'll be able to resolve those issues and put them behind us.

Unfortunately, what happens all too often is that people bail out of these relationships before they are able to resolve these conflicts. Why? "She drives me nuts! She's just like my mother!" Well, of course she is. That's partly why you chose her. You needed a stand-in for your mother at a peer level so you could conquer your feelings of powerlessness in relation to her. Instead, you see the similarities and bail on the relationship and your chance to finally get those issues with Mom resolved. The issues come up, it's painful, the person leaves. And they take that same unresolved issue into their next relationship. Of course, the chance of bailing out on that relationship when things get tough increases. Especially if you've chosen your mate on an impulsive whim because it was stimulating.

The irony is that we think we're looking for someone different from our parents. The logical thought is this: "I don't want to repeat my family history—the things I saw and grew up with. So I'm going to choose a mate who is very different from my parents." But on the subconscious level, we seek out people just like our parents so that we can get these issues resolved. Sometimes we actually manage to find someone who is very different from our parents. But all too often, when we do find them, we *force* them into the role of our parents by projecting onto them the very attributes we said we didn't want in a partner—attributes that partner doesn't really have but we need them to have so we can find resolution. Complicated stuff. Stuff most couples go through to some degree whether or not they have ADD. It's just a process in life most of us experience.

Let me give you an example. Lon and Sheri got married in their forties. They had both been through marriages that hadn't worked out, and Lon knew that his ADD contributed to the demise of his first and second marriages. This time, Lon and Sheri were committed to doing it right, committed to making the marriage work, and committed to each other. They were happy, they were in love, and they were sure they could make it all work out.

But the first time they had a real fight after they married, Lon panicked.

"I just felt totally defenseless," he told me. "I went back to this very early child ego state. In fact, after this humongous fight (verbal only), I went into the walk-in closet and lay down on the floor to go to sleep. I did that partly because I didn't know what else to do. And partly because I was afraid. I found myself lying there on the floor of the closet feeling very small and very young and very vulnerable. At the same time, I wondered what in the world I was doing there. Then Sheri came in and she felt so bad about the conflict. She apologized and told me not to worry and that everything would be okay."

Well, that part of the experience felt pretty good to Lon. He liked the fact that Sheri noticed the pain he was in and came to "take care of his pain." So the next time they had a big blowout, Lon went to the closet again, feeling and wondering the same things he felt the first time he had retreated there. And Sheri followed him there to apologize. But after a while, when Lon continued to go into the closet after every argument, Sheri got tired of following him. She caught on to his manipulation. She stopped coming in to rescue him. So there he was, a grown man, all alone in his closet.

"I finally realized that what I was doing was really dumb—I could feel it throughout my entire body, that sense of 'dumbness.' Sheri wasn't shaming me. And she wasn't buying in to the manipulation I subconsciously was attempting to make her see my pain and stop overpowering me with her anger the way my mom and dad overpowered me with their anger. She was just waiting for me and wondering what the heck I was doing in the closet. And all those old child-type issues of feeling shamed and defenseless and powerless were suddenly gone," he said. "That realization opened a path for me to understand a lot of other things in my life—issues I had been working on that developed while growing up. And I began to consider other areas of my life in which I was also acting more from a child's perspective than a grownup's. It was a huge turning point for me in my maturation as an adult and for our relationship. And since I experienced all of these things at a gut level, I really got it. I know I've really learned those lessons now."

Because people with ADD are kinesthetic learners, once they've learned a lesson through experience, they know they won't forget it. No one will ever be able to take that knowledge away from them once they have it kinesthetically.

The fact that Lon and Sheri are committed to their relationship in the deepest sense is the driving force that will help them get through future problems as well. And if that sense of commitment is missing, it is almost impossible to resolve the issues each of you bring with you into the relationship.

But it does take commitment.

5) The importance of resolving conflicts now.

For example, I recently worked with a couple that our clinical staff lovingly referred to as the "couple from hell." I saw this couple, both of whom had ADD, for psychotherapy, and a psychiatrist in our office was also following them medically. Because we often work together as a team, I would report my clinical impressions to this psychiatrist, who would then consider that information and make micro-adjustments in their medications to fine-tune the metabolic functioning in their brains. We worked at it, and worked at it, and worked at it. They kept coming back, but they continued to struggle—and they were downright miserable. Just the fact that they were consistently coming for counseling week after week told me that they really did want to work out their problems and once again fall—or rather, grow—in love all over again. They really wanted the relationship of their dreams and were willing to do whatever it took to make that happen. They had to commute an hour and a half—each way—to come to our clinic. The time, the distance, the consistency all spoke of their commitment. But they were absolutely miserable no matter how hard we all tried. But none of us ever gave up.

There was one week in particular when the psychiatrist adjusted both of their medications at the same time. He had been treating them for quite a while, and this wasn't the first time their medications had been changed. But this particular time, the micro-adjustment in their medications worked like a charm. The next time I saw them, they were a changed couple. It was amazing. They laughed together, smiled lovingly at each other, and were genuinely happy with each other—a huge difference from the preceding months. A huge difference from the preceding week.

I continued to meet with them for weekly therapy for another month. Each week the reports were the same. "Everything's great. We're doing fine." From the moment their medications were finally adjusted to the right dose for their brains, everything had changed. After the first month, we cut back on therapy to twice a month. Still, "Everything's great. We're doing fine." They had not had one single conflict in over six weeks. Prior to that their lives were a constant conflict. Now that both of them were able to better access their brains, they were able to use all the things that they had been working on in therapy and outside of therapy to try to make their relationship wonderful. Finally, they were back on a more stable course.

I saw this couple again after they had been on their new medications/doses for three months. They were genuinely warm toward each other. They were not fighting. They were straightening out the chaos in their lives, which was a result of their ADD-induced stress, and they are getting much better.

The last time I saw this couple in therapy, I asked them, "What was it that kept you two together when there was so much pain for both of you? What was the glue? In the midst of all that pain, how in the world did you stick with it?"

They both came back with the same answer—an answer which reflected a tremendous amount of thought on their part. They said, "We knew that if we didn't get it worked out here, it would just be the same with someone else. And we wanted to get these issues resolved once and for all so we could get on with our lives and have the romantic relationship with each other that we wanted so much."

Here were two very intelligent people, both ADD, who realized that, in addition to their metabolic problems, they had issues they had never resolved in any of their previous relationships—whether with their parents or other adult partners. And they knew these issues absolutely had to be resolved before either of them could move forward in their lives. We addressed their metabolic issues medically, and in therapy gave them the tools they needed (communication skills, boundary setting, alternate coping skills, etc.) to interact in a more positive manner. An accomplishment they might never have attained had they both given up on their commitment to work things out, "until death do us part."

It wasn't just psychotherapy that made them successful. They had been in psychotherapy before, and although it helped some, it hadn't made a huge difference. It wasn't just the medication therapy which was definitely needed. It was a combination of both medication therapy and psychotherapy that gave them the ability to be successful in their relationship. Today, they are a warm, loving, and supportive couple.

Although I believe completely in the value of commitment and the process of resolving old issues from childhood, not all relationships can be saved. And I want to be very, very clear that in some cases, the best thing you can possibly do is to get out of the relationship. Commitment is one thing—when both partners are stable and loving and mature. But commitment to a relationship that is harmful to one or both individuals is never a good idea.

If there is domestic violence occurring, or any kind of physical, sexual, or mental/emotional abuse, you need to physically get away. Find a safe place and see if you and your partner can work things out with a therapist or psychiatrist. When the relationship has deteriorated to that point, sometimes it can still be worked out. But safety always comes first. Get to a safe place and then do whatever you can to work things out without jeopardizing your safety. Therapy—psychological and medical—is usually a good way to help get back on track.

6) Fantasy projection.

People with ADD can be extremely creative. And along with that creativity comes an incredibly powerful and intellectually stimulating fantasy life. You may think that when we daydream we are totally out to lunch. But we've got an incredible fantasy life based on years of fantasy . . . or daydreaming, if you wish. Consequently, when someone with ADD meets someone new, or sees someone attractive across the room, they just might project their fantasy onto that person. Unfortunately, if we project our *fantasy* onto someone, we barely have room to see them for who they really are.

That might work fine as long as the relationship is stimulating. But all too often, when the honeymoon is over and the stimulation of newness dies down and the person with ADD finally sees their mate for who they really are, there's a terrible sense of disappointment.

Suddenly, you realize this person isn't who you thought he was. They lied to you. They pretended to be someone they weren't. They tricked you. They may have even trapped you into marriage. And you become angry at them. How could they do such a thing?

In reality, something very different happened. The non-ADD partner never lied to you, or tricked you or trapped you, or even pretended to be someone they weren't. They were themselves all along. But you didn't see them because you were so busy projecting your fantasy onto this real person. You never even gave yourself a chance to see them. But now that you've married them, you're taking a good long look at your mate—possibly for the very first time. You wake up some morning and turn to your mate in bed and ask them, "Who are you?" Unfortunately, you really mean it. Not the best way to start a life together—romantically involved with someone you've never really met because you projected your fantasy onto them. You've never seen and known them for who they really are.

So now we've seen all the pitfalls—everything that can (and too often does) go wrong in choosing a mate. Is there any way around it? Absolutely. Before we get started with the rest of the list, remember that this one thing supersedes all of the others: *If you have ADD, make certain you are on your medication(s) and followed closely by your physician.* You will make better choices in mate selection when your brain is working the way it is supposed to work.

Here are some questions to ask yourself as you're looking for Mr. or Ms. Right—someone you will be happy to wake up next to every day, even years after the honeymoon is over.

1. Were you friends first? The very best, most lasting, relationships begin with friendship and then move into a romantic friendship. It gives you a better chance of seeing the person for who they really are before you become blinded by love.

2. Are your friends or family telling you to take it slower? If the relationship is moving too fast—from introduction to living together or marriage—then you *are* probably moving too fast and it's time to put the brakes on a bit. If your friends are telling you there's a problem in the relationship or the way you're handling it, listen to them. They have an outsider's perspective that you need to take seriously. In the midst of new love, anyone's thinking can become clouded—more so if you have ADD. So listen to them and try to integrate their perspective into your understanding.

3. Are your friends or family telling you your boyfriend or girlfriend is less than wonderful? If so, try to listen objectively and see what they're really talking about instead of immediately becoming defensive and arguing.

4. Ask yourself this question: If this person never changes, do I want to spend the rest of my life with them just the way they are today?

5. If the person you are in love with has been diagnosed with ADD, are they taking their medication? Do they take it consistently? If not, are they working with a therapist to change some of the more destructive ADD behaviors?

6. If you suspect the person you're in love with has ADD, are they willing to have an evaluation? And if so, are they willing to take medication if they are diagnosed with ADD?

7. Is your partner willing to participate in couples premarital counseling—not necessarily because you already have problems, but to learn how to avoid them and develop the healthiest relationship possible?

If you're like most people and throw all caution to the wind to enjoy and savor every last drop of the endorphin release experienced by fantasy and hyperfocus on romance, go for the gusto. Just know that it won't last. And when you're ready . . . when you've had enough pain . . . seek the help of professionals to help you get your brain tuned up and to learn alternate coping skills so you can have the relationship of your dreams. It might take some work, but you deserve it.

What's the Best Combination for Success?

After I teach about ADD and Romantic Relationships at a conference or on our yearly cruise/seminar, I am often asked, "What's the best combination for a successful relationship? A partner with ADD and a partner without ADD? Or does a relationship have a better chance when both partners have ADD? And if they both have ADD, is it best for both to have the same type of ADD?"

After hearing all the possible problems of ADD in a romantic relationship, people understandably want to hedge their bets a little as they step up to the table and roll the dice in love and romance. But you are so much more than just your ADD. True, ADD can bring some frustration and pain to the relationship. But it can also bring some wonderful things as well. Things like creativity, intuition, spontaneity, fun, and yes, even wisdom born of years of pain.

You are both so much more than ADD or non-ADD. There are other aspects of who you are: your religious upbringing; your taste in music; the environment you grew up in; the kinds of friends you have; what your family was like; your level of education; where you were in your family birthing order. All of these things add up to a lot more than whether you are ADD or non-ADD.

So don't get all hung up about what the right combination is for you. The right combination for you is the one that works for both you and your partner. Even if you're a match made in heaven, without relationship tools and skills you've got a tough row to hoe ahead of you. And people who may not match up all that well in the first place can have a wonderful, loving life together if they have decent tools and skills in their relationship toolbox.

Scared? That's normal. Worried? Who isn't? Don't worry—I plan to equip you with even more tools for building the relationship of your dreams. First, however, we need to look at unrealistic expectations in romantic relationships.

▼▲▼▲▼▲▼▲

FOUR

▲▼▲▼▲▼▲▼

ADD and Unrealistic Expectations for Relationships

When relationships do not work out—whether or not ADD is involved—it's often because the expectations for that relationship were unrealistic in the first place.

For example, if you believe that marriage is a perpetual state of bliss in which your partner meets all of your needs on a daily basis, then you're bound to be unhappy in your marriage and unhappy with your mate. If you believe that when you find your one and only true love you will never be lonely or sad again, you're in for some rocky times. And if you believe that true love never involves differences of opinion or arguments, then prepare to be disappointed.

The best chance any relationship has for success comes when both parties are realistic about themselves, each other, and the relationship itself. When you know what you can reasonably expect, you're better prepared to deal with the difficult times that will come your way. And you're less likely to become so disheartened that you just want to give up altogether.

When ADD is involved, all of this becomes even more complicated. Because of their incredibly creative fantasy life (day-dreaming), people with ADD often aren't able to see their mate for who they really are. Instead, they see the *fantasy of their mate* which they've created in their mind. That unrealistic view of their partner can certainly increase the likelihood of having even more unrealistic expectations.

Plus, the non-ADD person will come into the relationship with their own set of unrealistic expectations. In terms of knowledge, there is what we know, what we don't know, and then . . . what we don't know we don't know. *That's* where things get interesting. Often that's the case for non-ADD people who connect with folks who have ADD. There may be a whole lot of "what you don't know you don't know" going on for a while.

Let's take a look at the seven most common unrealistic expectations people bring with them into relationships. As you will see, many of these things apply to relationships in which there is no ADD involved at all. But, when ADD is involved, some of the expectations get kicked up a few more notches.

How do you and your mate rate? Let's take a look and see.

1) "All you need is love."

Our pop culture inundates us with the message that all you really need to be happy in life is love. If only you have a boyfriend or girl-friend or husband or wife, the myth goes, and that person loves you enough and you love them enough, everything in your life will be great.

When you first fall in love and experience the rush of ecstatic happiness (endorphins), those feelings are so powerful and so positive that you want nothing more than to be by the side of your beloved so these intense, wonderful feelings can be available to both of you the rest of your lives. When you feel this wonderful, it can be hard to believe that anything could ever change.

That's how Tom and Betty felt when they first fell in love with each other during the first week on their new jobs. Both had been hired into the city planning department on the same day. Betty was an administrative assistant and Tom was a planning analyst. Their immediate attraction to each other was so strong it took them both by surprise. They had their first date the week they met, began dating each other exclusively the next month, were engaged within three months, and married within six. They were more in love than either of them could have believed possible. They just knew their happiness would last forever.

And it did last . . . for quite a while. Then Tom's mother, who lived in a small town about sixty miles away, became ill. After a few weeks, it became obvious that she could no longer live alone. Tom, her only son, wanted to do the right thing—the loving thing—and impulsively told her she could move in with him and Betty.

When Betty found out, she was absolutely furious. "How could you do this to me—to us?" she asked. "We never even talked about this as an option. Don't I have any say in the matter? After all, this is a marriage of two, not one! I can't take care of your mother and work full-time, too. Plus, now we're never going to have any privacy. I love your mother, but I can't believe you would make such a major decision without first consulting me!"

Tom was stunned by, and completely unprepared for, Betty's reaction. After all, this was his *mother*. What other choice did he have?

All you need is love? Not in this case. Tom and Betty really do love each other, but they need a lot more than love working for them at this moment. They need better communication and respect of boundaries, and they desperately need conflict resolution skills. Love alone just isn't enough.

Betty pinpointed the real problem in her comment that she and Tom had never even talked about his mother moving in with them. Which is true. That discussion never came up between the two of them. They truly believed (as many people mistakenly believe) that all you need is love. However, in real life, commitment and communication have to go along with it.

In this example we can see a major conflict which developed because Tom impulsively made a major decision which would have tremendous effect on both their lives without first discussing it with Betty. He just assumed she would understand and support him in his decision. Betty certainly had a legitimate reason to be angry. Betty loved Tom and Tom's mother. Most likely she would have fully supported the idea of her mother-in-law moving in with them. Her resistance was a result of not having been involved in the decision-making process. Tom's impulsive decision was forced upon her, and her sense of significance went right out the window. The feeling of "loss of significance" is very painful. When we look at conflict resolution skills in Chapter Nine, we'll learn more about the importance of significance in relationships and how to apply that concept to conflict resolution skills. For now, just be aware of the importance of significance, as it will be a recurring theme throughout this book. This concept is vitally important to having a successful romantic relationship.

Our popular culture shows us that real-life problems like the one Tom and Betty are working through—having a sick relative move in unexpectedly—can be resolved in thirty minutes or less. Problems get resolved that quickly all the time on TV sitcoms. But sitcoms are not reality. In the real world, we must have realistic expectations about marriage, and our partner, in order for the relationship to endure. The latter is especially true in a relationship involving ADD.

Both partners in an ADD-affected relationship need to have realistic expectations of each other. They need to learn as much as they can about ADD and non-ADD behaviors. It is not an equal relationship if only the non-ADD person is forced into understanding and accepting ADD behaviors. Granted, knowing and understanding ADD behaviors will help to diminish their unrealistic expectations of their ADD spouse. But the person who has ADD also needs to learn from their partner and/or therapist about the non-ADD person's view of life, to better understand how their ADD behaviors affect the people they love. They also need to learn how non-ADD people "do" life. ADD and non-ADD are two very different approaches to life. When both partners understand both sides of the fence, they can then have more realistic expectations about each other.

So having realistic expectations is very important. Clearly, in order to have a successful relationship, you need a lot more than love. You also need tools.

To build a strong foundation for a lifetime of love, commitment is another tool you'll both need. People with ADD often have a difficult time staying on task. This is also true in terms of staying on task with a commitment—even in a romantic relationship. That's certainly not true for everyone with ADD, but it can be a problem.

As we discussed in Chapter Two, people with ADD have a need for constant stimulation. They understand life through their kinesthetic experience of life. Once the excitement and stimulation of new love wears off in the relationship, the ADD person may become panicked or distant. When the newness of the relationship wears off, the person with ADD most likely will experience a decrease in biochemical stimulation, the endorphins experienced as a result of the new love experience. That biochemical change, experienced kinesthetically, changes their understanding of the relationship—drastically. They may doubt their judgment in having chosen you as their partner. They may feel trapped—terrified that they are now locked into a situation in which they will suffocate and die from lack of stimulation. They honestly don't feel well in their own bodies at this time. Because of this, they may seek stimulation elsewhere. It may be that the ADD person ends up like Martin (in Chapter Two) who hyperfocused on romance, then sailboats, then hockey—and who knows what's next.

The ADD person may move from relationship to relationship as an outward manifestation of their need for constant stimulation. They may also have an unrealistic expectation of finding the "perfect mate"—never-ending love (lots of stimulation) with someone who will keep them charged up biochemically. In essence, they'll know when they find the right mate because they will *feel* it in their body . . . and that feeling will then last a lifetime. It's a wonderful idea, but unrealistic.

There's more at play here than just ADD. Family values, cultural norms, and individual personalities all affect how the ADD person will gravitate towards stimulation. As a result of this, some ADD folks learn how to find stimulation in more appropriate ways than others, such as through stimulating challenges at work; creative processes in hobbies and crafts; sports; or church. But regardless of whether they do it appropriately or inappropriately, they *will* find ways to activate their prefrontal cortex. It is either do or die. After a string of failed romantic relationships people with ADD may give up on love altogether and subconsciously also give up on getting the stimulation they need, they become demoralized and depressed. If the depression is significant enough, it may culminate in taking their own life.

Commitment—staying on task in the relationship, regardless of how you feel—is the glue that holds the relationship together. True, we maintain our commitment out of love for our partner. But ask anyone who's been married for a long time. That person will tell you there were plenty of times throughout their romantic relationship when they became thoroughly disenchanted with their partner. Out of their *commitment* (not intense feelings of love) they worked through the difficulties they faced in life—whether it was an ill parent moving in to live with them, child-rearing differences, or financial difficulties. Love was definitely not enough when it came to facing tough times together.

Good communication—communication that travels in both

directions, is respectful, and is understood by both partners—is another major tool in maintaining a lifelong romantic relationship. Without good communication, a couple is likely to face a lifetime of lunacy instead of a lifetime of love. All of Chapter Five is devoted to learning about communication, because good communication is of tantamount importance for a relationship to flourish and thrive.

All you need is love? It certainly sounds right, but in reality, love is just never enough by itself. After all, even the Beatles broke up—shortly after their song, "All You Need Is Love," became a huge hit.

2) "Now that we're married, everything should settle down and it will be smooth sailing from here on out."

Where do we get these crazy ideas? We certainly don't get them from anyone we know. Have you ever seen a couple who was married for a long period of time who didn't have problems that needed to be worked out?

Think about your parents, your aunts and uncles, your friends, your co-workers. Every couple has some kind of issue or problem that really needs to be worked out. That's just part of life. It might not involve the illness of a family member, but everyone has problems to solve. You will always have challenges to face together as a couple. That's life. How the two of you face those problems together has a great deal to do with the quality of your relationship.

Who's going to do the housework? Cook the meals? Balance the checkbook? Are you going to have children? If you do, are both parents going to work? How in the world are you going to pay all the bills this month? These kinds of things are real-life issues and problems that couples will have to face. "Now that we're married it will be smooth sailing from here on out?" Actually, your struggles are just beginning as the two of you learn to live together in harmony. Hopefully you will learn from each other, with both changing, both growing. Commitment is the glue that holds a relationship together through the process of learning, changing, and growing. A process which, oftentimes, can be very painful and scary.

People who want to stay married for the long haul have to be willing to face, and work on, tough problems. In order to accomplish this, the relationship itself has to be cared for and nourished.

There are many ways in which romantic relationships are nourished. Think back to the beginning of the relationship. Remember all the time you spent with your partner doing things the two of you enjoyed? Remember sending mushy greeting cards and stealing moments on the phone at work just to say "I love you"? Walks on the beach, long conversations over romantic dinners, camping, snuggling in front of the TV, sharing your thoughts and feelings over a cup of coffee—those are just some of the many, many activities that nourish and replenish romantic relationships.

But all too often those intimate activities fall by the wayside. If you want to keep your relationship alive and vibrant, you can't replace all of those "together" activities with individual interests, a second job, caring for children, individual hobbies, individual civic interests. Regardless of what those activities are—and they certainly have value—they are not "together" activities.

You need those "together" moments—the very activities that caused your relationship to blossom and grow in the first place—in order to nourish your relationship as it matures. That way, you'll be prepared to weather life's storms as a team. You'll be able to count on the strength of your love to sustain you when the sailing gets rough. And you'll also have a lot more fun.

In many ways, relationships are organic and must be nourished and cared for, almost like any other living thing, in order to grow. If not, they will predictably wither and die. You know this is true for other organic entities. Your challenge is to value and respect your romantic relationship as if it had a life of its own, and treat it accordingly.

For example, suppose you go to a grocery store and see row after row of beautiful plants in wicker baskets. As a person who enjoys the beauty of live plants, you buy one and take it home. And just as you had imagined, it looks wonderful there in a corner of your kitchen.

After a while, you notice that your plant is wilting, but you don't do anything about it. You just hope that it will start looking good again soon. You hope and hope and hope it will perk up. You even pray that God will breathe life back into this poor dying plant. But eventually the plant looks worse and worse until it dies—and then there is no other recourse but to throw it out.

How dare that plant die! You invested your hard-earned money in it. You brought it home. You loved that plant and had hopes for it to grow and thrive and add to the enjoyment of your life.

All of the above may be true, but *you never actively took care of it.* You never watered it or fed it or took it out into the sunshine. You loved that plant, but you didn't nurture it. And so it died.

Relationships are exactly like that. The wonderful feelings of love we have at the beginning of relationships are very important. We want those feelings and we need them. Our love seems to be in full blossom and we love every minute of it. But after the honeymoon phase is over—and it will end for everyone at some point in a romantic relationship—you have to actively nurture your relationship if you want it to thrive.

3) "I've met the most wonderful guy. Finally. Someone who can meet all of my needs."

Granted, it is unlikely that anyone would actually make a statement quite like that in these enlightened times. But even so, this third mistaken expectation is woven into the fabric of many people's minds—male and female alike. And there is an increase of this when ADD is involved. Many people hope that their partners will help them compensate for their ADD behaviors and will always be there for them, every second of every day. Someone who will always love and accept them regardless of how stressful their ADD behaviors may be to their spouse. Someone to rescue them from their pain. The "perfect" spouse or lover. It is unrealistic to believe that our mate will be able to meet our every need.

When we're little kids going through the developmental process, we form an understanding of our world through the information we receive. Kids hear lots and lots of fairy tales while growing up. And they witness the actions of their parents, who have internalized the fairy tales *they* heard while they were growing up. Then we see those same fairy tales played out before our very eyes in movies and on TV. Although we know they're fairy tales, we have still come to believe in them at some very deep level. Probably because we always want and need for the good guys to win. Probably because they feed the magical, simplistic thinking of a child. And these stories are very stimulating.

Take Cinderella, for example. Her family is emotionally distant and cruel. Her work is monotonous. She's feeling hopeless. (ADD people often feel hopeless.) But then one day a handsome young prince comes and, with the help of her fairy godmother and a stylish pair of slippers, rescues her from her drudgery and escorts her into a brand-new life filled with love and luxury.

You get the picture. Whether it's fairy tales, animated cartoons, or Barbie's dream house, little girls are still sold a bill of goods in our culture. And the message to them is that their own special Prince Charming will come along and rescue them from all their problems.

Men often grow up with similar myths based on the same fairy tales. That they are to be gallant. Charming. Loving. Constant. Altruistic. Invincible. Omnipotent. Then we each try to act out our parts just as the script was written. Except of course, none of it works very well—especially for those of us with ADD. Personally, I had to trade in my Prince Charming hat a long time ago. To perform in life as a real Prince Charming would be difficult for anyone.

For someone with ADD, it is flat-out impossible! The more we try to play our role, the crazier things get in the relationship because we just can't be that Prince guy.

And the same is true for grownup little girls needing someone to rescue them from the entrapment they feel in their own ADD life—Mr. "Prince ADD Charming." Whoever she puts into that role in her life, no matter who he is, will soon be shattering her dreams.

Another mistaken belief is thinking our partner will just naturally be interested in the same things we're interested in. So Bill naturally believes his wife will come to thoroughly enjoy tinkering with old farm engines. Or Fran is just certain that her husband, once he gets the knack of it, will be as enthralled as she is with propagating African violets. That way, they won't have to turn anywhere else to have their needs fulfilled in terms of shared interests. Their partner will always be there to meet their every need in friendship and camaraderie.

In reality, of course, it's ludicrous for them to believe that their partner will want to do everything they want to do. Or that she will take the place of male friends in his life. Or that he will take the place of female friends in her life. Of course, they're both likely to have some mutual interests, but they'll still have a need for outside friendships and individual interests. Neither can fulfill all of their mate's needs. It's just impossible. To attempt such a feat creates a closed system which excludes input or output from other life experiences.

Closed systems are like ponds of water which sit alone without fresh water moving in and old water moving out. They become stagnant, stinking, and toxic to life. The same is true of relationships in which the partners meet each other's every need. After a while, the relationship becomes stagnant and toxic.

This is all very true for people with or without ADD. But when one or both of the partners in a relationship has ADD, these unrealistic expectations can be exacerbated. Because people with ADD often have a very rich fantasy life, they are sometimes not realistic in understanding who their partner really is. That makes it even easier to project their own interests and desires onto that person— and see their mate through the eyes of their fantasy.

Bradley, who has ADD, may miss the fact that his wife, Melissa, has absolutely no interest in tennis, for which he has a passion. Melissa probably didn't give him any reason to think she shared that passion. But in Bradley's initial love and rapture for her, he imagined she would just naturally love tennis. After all, what's not to love? It's a great game that millions of people enjoy. And although Melissa might enjoy the sport, Bradley trudged through the courting process without first finding out whether she has any interest in the sport or if she hates the game. Bradley never found out *who she really is* as opposed to his *fantasy* of who she is.

We are all complex people with many interests and many needs. No one person can ever meet all of those needs. That's absolutely normal. But when we expect that in a relationship, we are setting ourselves up for disappointment, pain, and possibly even failure.

Some of the most common unrealistic expectations that couples face, when ADD is involved, are related to ADD behaviors and apologies for those behaviors. The ADD person may expect their mate to totally understand them and therefore absolve them when they make mistakes. They want their partner to fill their need to be understood. That's not a bad thing at all. We would all like to be understood by our mates. But that unrealistic expectation means they feel trampled upon when their partner is angry with them for some ADD mistake. Like impulsively saying something that was demeaning to their partner, or bouncing a series of checks because there wasn't enough money in the checking account. Or bringing the boss home for dinner without first checking their partner's plans for the night. And when the ADD person screws up, they often believe their partner will gracefully forgive them. "Wait a minute! I've got ADD and that's why it happened. You're supposed to understand and forgive me, not be angry with me! What's up with you? You're supposed to meet my every need—especially love and acceptance when I've done something that hurts you. After all, I said I was sorry!"

The ADD person further hurts their spouse by defending themselves rather than accepting that the consequences of their behavior have somehow hurt their partner. That defensive move further hurts their partner because it undermines their sense of significance.

The non-ADD person has a similar problem. They unrealistically expect their impulsive ADD partner to not say or do things impulsively. That's like expecting a fish to not swim. They expect their partner to be and think like them . . . the way non-ADD people think and act. So when their ADD partner makes a mistake that's a result of their ADD, they become infuriated because it was a thoughtless thing to do. They take it as a personal attack on them rather than seeing it for what it is, ADD behavior. It's as if they want to throw the baby out with the bath water. Understandably, living with ADD can be very frustrating at times. People with ADD often exhibit behaviors—because of the physical limitations of their brain metabolism—that are difficult to live with. But those behaviors, which are often inappropriate, are not meant with malice. To unrealistically expect an ADD partner to not act ADD will only increase the frustration level.

This doesn't mean that people with ADD shouldn't be held accountable for their actions. Knowing that you are ADD is never an excuse for inappropriate behaviors. It is your responsibility to get the help you need—both medical and behavioral—so that you can function appropriately in your relationships. ADD might be a cause, but it should never be used or tolerated as an excuse.

Unrealistic expectations for the relationship, for your partner, and for your lives together will frustrate you both. As the two of you learn how to live and work together you will likely find all kinds of areas where you have held unrealistic expectations. That's okay. Use those experiences as a way to learn more about each other, expand your knowledge, and become more whole and complete. The more realistic your expectations become, the more likely you'll be able to create compensating skills to improve the quality of your relationship.

4) "I know she has some problems. But she'll change if I just love her enough."

Let's look at another way fairy tales have influenced our thinking about relationships.

Remember Belle from the classic French fairy tale, Beauty and the Beast? The man who wants to marry her doesn't interest her at all. Although he pursues her, Belle goes after someone else, a misunderstood guy who looks like he needs a bit of mothering and help—the Beast (okay, this guy needs a lot of help). Of course, Belle knows just how to take care of him, with a love that is true and pure. And when the Beast sees how much she loves him, he immediately changes into the man she's been waiting for—and a Prince to boot! Out of her powerful, healing love, she now has a brand-new life filled with love and contentment.

This is the woman who sees all the "possibilities" in the man she will marry, and what she can do to help him really reach his potential. Now *there's* a job with some serious stimulation, magical thinking, and a glorious outcome. The lesson we learn as children is: no matter how bad it gets (a Beast, no less), "I'll just make my own Prince Charming!" But after the marriage drags on for a while, she finds she has taken on an impossible task: making the irritable, often stuck-in-his-thinking, impulsive "man of her dreams" into a non-ADD Prince. That's enough to make anyone weary. And what an unfair way to choose a mate in the first place—"I love you, not for who you are, but for who I can mold you into being." This approach certainly will frustrate her to no end, exhaust her limited supply of energy and really, really anger her would-be Prince.

It's important to realize that this concept of loving someone enough for them to change their behavior is at the very heart of codependency. It's grandiose thinking to believe that your love is so powerful that it's not only enough for you, but it will be enough to "fix" the other person, too. And while we're at it . . . who made you God in the first place? Who gave you the sovereign right to try to change your partner?

In reality, that type of thinking is absolutely ludicrous. Yes, it is possible for your partner to change, but only if they want to make that change for their own personal reasons. Your love will never be enough to effect that change, in and of itself.

Warren is married to an artist with ADD, predominately inattentive type. She is not hyper or impulsive but does have attention problems. He knew Maggie had ADD when they first met because she told him. He knew she had difficulty following through with tasks. He knew that she was nowhere near reaching her potential as an artist. He knew that she was not a good communicator, and often he had to guess at what she was feeling or wanting.

Maggie was raised in an ADD and alcoholic family—her dad was ADD, impulsive type, and a raging alcoholic. He often made mean and discouraging comments to her. Years and years of verbal and emotional abuse had taken their toll on Maggie's self-esteem and self-image.

Warren knew all of these things but "loved her so much" he chose to ignore them. "She has so much potential," he would tell himself. "If I can just get her past that stuff, she will be incredible. What she really needs is love. If I just love her enough, my love will help to heal her childhood scars."

I've met Maggie and I know why Warren became so attached to her. She is a genuinely nice person and very attractive. And

Warren was right, she has a tremendous amount of potential that she has not tapped into yet. Were she to access her potential, she could really skyrocket as a human, as an artist, and as a mate. But Warren was wrong in making Maggie his personal project in life—believing that his love for her could change her into that model of success. He assumed that if he just showed Maggie enough love, everything would turn out all right. If he could just love her enough to heal all of those old childhood scars, she would be healed and grow and blossom. It wasn't just that Warren loved Maggie, she was also his personal project to work on. If he were successful, he would then have validation that he too is valuable. He needed Maggie to be someone who could not reach her potential, so he could fix her. Then *he* would be okay.

Unfortunately, this describes codependent behavior to a "T." Warren needed Maggie to be ADD so he could fix her. Then she, out of gratitude, would always love him for making her a success. That sense of owing would be the glue that kept them together, because Warren believed deep down inside that he could never have someone in his life as wonderful and beautiful as Maggie unless she owed him in some way. He didn't feel he really deserved her. These beliefs were working in Warren at a subconscious level. He was unconscious of these motivations—as are most people when they choose a mate to be their "project" instead of their partner. It's possible that Warren also has ADD and has chosen Maggie as his lifelong project because the challenge of fixing her is very stimulating for him. He'll always have somebody to hyperfocus on for stimulation.

Of course, the outcome of such a relationship is dismal. It's not a real romantic relationship, although both believe it is.

Maggie was happy to have found someone who "loved" her so much, but she couldn't allow herself to feel worthy of that love. This worked out great for Warren. Since she had become his project for life, he would have to make certain that she never really got better. If he really was able to fix her, she'd leave him. So, in essence, he had to prevent her from reaching her potential.

Although Maggie felt Warren's actions were loving, she also felt as if something was wrong, as if Warren was manipulating her in some way. She just couldn't put her finger on what it was. He said and did all these "loving" things. Still, something felt strange to her. He always seemed to be in a dominant position, which made her feel as if she was in a submissive one. Warren does love Maggie, but his motivations are very confused. It's no wonder then that Maggie feels something is wrong between them and starts to subconsciously put distance between them as a way to protect herself.

You may think you can change someone—love them into wholeness—but seldom does this fantasy become reality.

So what do you do when you love each other but ADD is involved, as it is in Warren and Maggie's situation?

Let's say the person you're in love with is basically sloppy (an ADD characteristic) and that really bothers you. You'd better be prepared to spend the rest of your life with a sloppy person and accept loving that person, sloppy and all, if you're going to marry them. That person is probably not going to change. Why? Because that just may be part of who they are.

Likewise, if you're a sloppy person and are entertaining thoughts of marrying someone who is very tidy, you could be looking at an unrealistic match. Sloppy or tidy really doesn't matter. Neither lifestyle is inherently wrong. There are plenty of wonderful people out there who are wonderfully sloppy. And there are plenty of wonderful people out there who are wonderfully tidy. That's not the point. If you're choosing to live with that person the rest of your life, you'd both better be comfortable living with someone who is completely the opposite of you in terms of tidy/sloppy.

Let's say you are a night owl, as many ADD folks can be, and your partner is a morning kind of guy. You'd better ask yourself, right now, if you can deal with that biological discrepancy. If something as basic as the time you eat dinner is important to you, you'd better work it out now. Because the chance of someone else coming around to your time schedule may end up as a lesson in futility. If the issue isn't really very important to your partner, they might be willing to change to accommodate you, but it doesn't happen often.

If your partner has lots of potential which they're not reaching, that better be okay with you. Love means accepting your partner the way that they are in this moment, loving them in this moment, because that's all you really have, anyway. Tomorrow may never come. If you love only what your partner has the potential of becoming, then you don't really love *them*, you love your fantasy.

Loving a fantasy is neither fair to your partner nor to you. It's not a love based in reality. Reality is who your partner is *right now*. This does not mean that you will always agree, that you will like every little thing about your lover. It does mean that you accept the good with the bad. There is no such thing as the perfect mate. If your mate should change on their own, in ways that you like, that's a gift. It's not something you have a right to expect.

As if Warren trying to change Maggie wasn't damaging enough, this type of thinking also puts unrealistic expectations on Warren, too. Not only is Warren sick at heart that Maggie is not living up to her potential as an artist, and struggles with intimacy issues associated with being an adult child of an alcoholic, he is also dealing with *his* feelings of failure stemming from his inability to "cure" her. If he had been more knowledgeable and realistic about the situation he faced, he would never have expected his love for Maggie to be able to perform impossible miracles.

Warren was misinformed and misguided, but in some ways, his motives were pure. He genuinely loved Maggie and wanted to help her. When Warren said "until death do us part," he meant it. Fortunately, Warren is now learning how to let go with love rather than trying to manipulate Maggie into changing. Amazingly, they are both finally beginning to see changes in Maggie—changes that could not happen until Warren was able to let go of his need to change Maggie and learn how to accept her the way she really is. That in and of itself was very healing for Maggie. Finally there was someone who saw her with all her warts and blemishes and loved her anyway. Loved her for her heart, not for the image she tried so hard to maintain. An image she thought necessary for people to find her lovable.

There are people who can only feel good about themselves when they are "fixing" other people. It gives them a feeling of power (stimulation), which is the only way they seem to be able to build any sense of self-esteem—by being able to fix someone else. The connotation to this is that they are more powerful and complete than the person they are attempting to change. The subconscious message behind their behavior is, "If I can pull this off, then I will have earned their love. They will love and appreciate me because of what I have done for them." The "changer" is afraid that they are not lovable the way they are. That they have to prove themselves worthy of someone else's affection. Warren began the relationship this way but is now learning to love Maggie in more healthy ways.

People with ADD can easily fall into the trap of trying to "fix" their partner because a person with ADD has a tendency to over-focus. Once he or she latches onto the concept of changing their partner, it's difficult for them to let go of it. They make changing their partner their all-encompassing task. Their project. Their assignment. They become completely focused on their partner and their problems. Why? Because they are stimulated by the challenge of trying to "fix" their partner, and in that sense the whole process actually becomes their medication—the stimulation their brain needs so they can feel better in their own body.

To use your partner as your neurostimulant in this fashion is a very inappropriate use of a partner. On the surface it may look like love. You may even believe that what you are doing is loving, but your motivation is way out of whack.

In terms of ADD and codependency, there are three different possible combinations: 1) the ADD person overfocused on changing their partner, 2) the non-ADD partner trying to change the ADD person, and 3) both partners trying to change each other. Regardless of who is responsible for the codependent behavior, believing that enough "love" will change your partner into a "super mate" is ludicrous and will frustrate both of you.

5) "It's not my fault."

Whenever we envision a relationship, generally we think about the good things. We know what will be great—the sharing, the closeness, the fun, and the sexual intimacy, to name a few. We also give a wink and a nod to the concept of "We'll have our share of problems along the way, just like any other couple," though we rarely have any idea of what we're *really* in for, which is probably best. "I know I'm not perfect," we might say, as a way to intellectually concede that we may be personally contributing to the struggles we're experiencing.

People with ADD have a greater tendency to deny the consequences of their imperfections. They often blame their beloved for the difficulties in the relationship rather than admit their part in creating them. This happens for a couple of reasons. First, ADD people have been accused of inappropriate behavior all of their life. After a while they develop an ego defense—a way to protect their self-esteem and self-concept—which denies any responsibility for the consequences of their behaviors. This way they can still see themselves as a good person. Second, they believe they are intelligent, so they deny any perspective different from their own. Their perspective must be the right one.

So they think they're right and then expect their partner to come to them and apologize for whatever it is they did wrong. Through this process, they have protected their ego. They are now safe from ridicule—the kind of ridicule they have experienced for years. As the fantasy continues, they believe that their partner will be impressed with their intelligence and automatically love and respect them even more.

It makes sense in a convoluted way. Unfortunately, in the process of protecting their damaged ego by blaming the "love of their life," the result is *less* respect. Out of their need to be right, they inadvertently make their partner wrong. They damage the relationship, and the morale and esteem of their mate.

Many times when I couldn't find something I was looking for my first thought was, "Terri must have taken it or moved it without telling me where she put it." I've even accused my wife of doing such a thing. Usually, I was the one who had misplaced the item because I wasn't paying attention to where I was and what I was doing the last time the item was in my hands. It wasn't my wife, it was me and my ADD.

Objectively, of course, we know that no one can be right all the time. But one of the most damaging and unrealistic assumptions we bring to relationships is the concept that we would never do anything to damage the relationship, because we love our partner. If we have an argument about something it's got to be because *they just don't understand us*. Wrong. Owning up to our part in a conflict, instead of projecting blame on our partner, requires the ability to consider perspectives we may have never considered before—specifically, our partner's. Not an easy task if you get stuck in your thinking or if you're mainly a kinesthetic learner.

If we're feeling sad or lonely, rather than asking ourselves what *we* are doing to create that experience, we instead focus on trying to figure out what our *partner* was or wasn't doing that made us feel that way.

Veronica thinks: "Sex isn't as satisfying as it should be. He's not doing this the way I like it." Adam thinks: "If she'd just relax a little more, sex would be a lot more fun." Both are blaming the other instead of taking responsibility to make certain they both get what they want and need sexually. It's so easy to get caught up in some ridiculous idea of right and wrong and totally miss the real issue: making certain both partners are getting their needs met. That, by far, is much more important than who's right or who's wrong. And it's a lot more mutually satisfying than winning an argument.

Let me give you a real-life example to show you what I'm talking about. I know an ADD couple who have been married for over twenty years and are basically happy together. But there's this one problem that keeps coming up over and over again: time.

Gene likes to be on time. It's a matter of personal pride to him and understandably so. As a child, being punctual had been a real problem for him because of his ADD. His father was very demanding about punctuality. So Gene worked very hard at forcing himself to be punctual, and he was successful at making that change. And just like his dad, Gene came to expect other people to be punctual.

Loraine is a little more relaxed about time. She tries to be on time because she knows how important it is to Gene, and she does a pretty good job. But occasionally, when her ADD kicks in on a day when there are lots of things to distract her from keeping track of the time and staying on task, she may run a little bit behind.

This last year, as a way to celebrate their twentieth wedding anniversary, Gene and Loraine decided on a four-day cruise. The ship was to leave the dock at eight o'clock at night. Gene said he wanted them to leave the house at 6:30 so they could board the ship by seven at the latest. Fortunately, they live fairly close to the harbor, so they'd have plenty of time to get there and relax for a while before they set sail on their personal "love boat."

Unfortunately, Loraine was having one of those days when her ADD was running in high gear. She didn't get home until 6:50 that evening. Gene was pacing. He didn't say anything, but she knew he was angry. They both grabbed their luggage and, in silence, rushed off to catch the ship. Because they live so close to the harbor, despite the late start they were still parked and on board the ship by about 7:20. More than a half hour to spare. Gene was still angry and stayed angry the entire night. They had a "lovely" dinner—in silence. They went to the show that night and saw one of their favorite comedians. Neither one of them talked. And although the jokes were funny, neither one of them laughed. Not once. Loraine was so self-conscious about the tension between them, she was certain everyone around them knew they were quarreling.

When they finally got back to their cabin, Loraine couldn't take it anymore. "What's the matter with you?" she cried. "This is our anniversary. We're supposed to be having a good time!"

"What's the matter with me? What's the matter with you? You knew we were supposed to leave the house by 6:30. You didn't even show up until ten minutes before seven. This is all your fault, you know! You ruined the whole evening, Loraine. Thanks a lot!"

Sounds like there's trouble in paradise. Gene was moody and sullen that whole night—absolutely convinced that it was Loraine who had ruined the first night of their anniversary cruise. He was so stuck in his need for punctuality that he couldn't let go. He fumed the whole night. Both of them were miserable, and each had a part in this fiasco. Loraine for running late and Gene for not letting go of his punctuality expectations. Neither of them was getting what they wanted: to have a lovely evening celebrating their anniversary. That went right out the door when "who's right/who's wrong" became the issue. Consequently, they were both miserable.

For a relationship to really flourish and do well, it's imperative that both partners be willing to see how they get stuck in "who's right/who's wrong" thinking and exchange that for "let's do whatever we need to make certain that we each get our needs met."

6) "If he would just take his medicine, everything would be fine!"

As we discussed in Chapter Two, ADD is a medical problem. Consequently, medication is most often the first line of defense for ADD, with additional interventions such as counseling and

93

therapy used in conjunction with the medication. I have seen many, many people with ADD whose lives have been turned around in very positive ways just through the use of prescription medication.

If you have problems in a relationship because of ADD, you need to be aware that medication is seldom the complete answer to those problems. All the medicine does is help the brain work more like it's supposed to work by increasing specific neurotransmitters. There are plenty of people whose brains work great without medication and are still in some messed-up romantic relationships. Just because your brain starts to work better is no guarantee the relationship is going to get better. Medication is only one tool in the treatment of ADD. There are lots of other tools and skills you will most likely need if you are to have the relationship of your dreams—one that will grow and blossom over a lifetime together. We all need a wide variety of skills and tools to achieve meaningful lives and lasting relationships, and you can't get those skills from any pill.

Think of it like this: Suppose you were extremely farsighted from birth and for some reason your vision was never corrected. And let's also suppose you found yourself fascinated with fashion design and wanted to learn to sew. Unfortunately, with your vision problem, sewing would not be in the cards for you. No matter how badly you truly wanted to learn to sew, you just would not be able to get that slim piece of thread through the eye of the needle. You wouldn't have been able to decipher the markings on the sewing machine or the shirt pattern, either.

Now let's suppose that your vision was suddenly corrected when you were twenty years old. Suddenly you were able to see things you'd never seen before. You could read fine print. You could see the eye of the needle for the first time. Great!

But does that mean you would know how to sew? Would you suddenly know how to make a button hole or a placket for a zipper? I don't think so. Just because you were able to see the smallest parts of a sewing machine clearly for the first time doesn't mean you would have any idea how to sew. You might have gained the physical ability—but you wouldn't immediately have the knowledge or skill to go with it.

It's the same with ADD. We may go undiagnosed and untreated for years. And there are all kinds of social skills, interpersonal relationship skills, and communication skills that we just didn't learn completely while we were growing up. Our brains just weren't working for us well enough. Then someone comes up to us and says: "Hey, you've got ADD. Why don't you go get an evaluation and get some medication so you can function better?" So we do just that and our physician puts us on medication. You know what? We still don't have the social skills we missed growing up. Why? Because even though our brains are working better with medication, we still have to learn the things we missed growing up when our brains weren't working at capacity.

Medication usually doesn't make things better instantly. In fact, it's a rare occurrence for adults to have a huge, enlightening experience when they start medication. It does happen, but it's not the norm. The longer they've been on medication the more change they and their partner will probably see. It's just like the farsighted fellow we just talked about, except this time it wasn't a visual disability, it was a neurobiological one.

But there is yet another angle to how medication may affect the relationship.

In some situations, when the ADD partner begins taking medication, the relationship actually takes a turn for the worse. When an individual starts medication, changes begin to take place. That's what we were hoping for in the first place, right? But as they begin to change, their partner might notice that they are becoming someone different from the person they married. Sirens and bells go off in their partner's head: "Danger, danger, danger. Something is different here. Something is changing. This is upsetting the status quo. This is scary!"

In all probability, the ADD partner will be somewhat easier to get along with after starting medication. They may be able to better communicate with their partner. They may have better impulse control and be more present in the relationship. These changes are not changes in their personality. They are still who they were all along. They just couldn't access what they needed to communicate better, show greater impulse control, and be more present. A lot of people are afraid of taking medications for ADD because they're afraid it will alter their personality. Yes, there will be changes. But these changes only affect how their brain functions. The basics of who they are, the person they are deep down in their soul, doesn't change. That stays constant. All in all, if the medication is working correctly, the change is about getting better, becoming more whole and complete. Becoming more of who they really are. Yes, thank God, they will be changing.

Sometimes these changes can cause problems in romantic relationships. For example, sometimes a person with ADD can have trouble expressing his or her feelings. After taking medication the ADD person can now suddenly express the feelings they had been keeping inside. That can be a terrific thing—as long as those feelings are pleasant. What happens to the relationship if the person with ADD has hurt and angry feelings which have been there all along, but were inaccessible? Now the person is able to access and express those feelings for the first time. For the non-ADD partner, this can be an extremely difficult paradigm shift. After all, they have never seen their partner get really angry before. And it can be even more difficult if that anger is directed at the non-ADD person.

Shirley had begged Buddy to share his feelings with her for years. At one point she even considered leaving the relationship for lack of emotional intimacy. But she stayed. Eventually Buddy was diagnosed as having ADD and placed on medication. He started to feel. The only problem for Shirley was that her husband was not only sharing close intimate feelings, he was also expressing anger. Shirley was not used to having Buddy angry with her. This was new . . . and scary.

Did Buddy's personality change? Not really. Finally, he had access to his feelings—all of them—love, hurt, joy, sadness, and yes, even anger.

Whenever one person in a relationship changes, that will have some effect on the other person in the relationship. Whether or not these changes will be viewed as good or bad depends on each individual's ability to adjust to change.

And that brings us back to why commitment in a relationship is so important. If we're really committed to the relationship, then we hang in there with our partners—even when they go through their changes and adjustments.

Change is difficult, and most of us are frightened of change. I know one couple in which the wife, Freda, stated—vehemently— that she liked her husband, Jose, better before he started his ADD medication. She didn't like the changes at all. But Jose did. On medication, he was able to become more of who he really is. Now he was leading a more active life. Jose was developing hobbies and other interests. Prior to this, he would come home from work, sit on the couch, and watch that day's recorded soap operas with Freda until it was time to go to bed. Freda was a very depressed woman and wanted Jose to stay there all night, every night, watching the soaps with her. Until diagnosis and medication of his ADD, he was willing to do just that because he thought he had to give up doing any of the things he liked so he could codependently take care of her.

This was extremely difficult for Freda because she had grown used to the pattern of her husband going to work every day, then coming home and watching TV with her—not that that's necessarily bad. But now he was developing other interests in life—interests that had always been there but that he couldn't pursue because he had become very codependent with his wife. Now that his brain was working better, he realized that he didn't care to watch soap operas. He felt that he was missing out on a lot of life. Now he was going out to see friends after work. He spent time working on the snowmobiles that had sat in their garage for over ten years after they traded snowmobiling for soaps. Jose would offer to take Freda out, encourage her to go with him to see friends, talk about taking a snowmobile trip like they used to. But she just wanted to stay home and watch her soap operas . . . and she wanted him to stay at home with her to watch them.

The changes he made as a result of medication—positive changes for him—certainly caused problems in the relationship. She didn't like her "new" husband. He wasn't exactly what she had planned on spending the rest of her life with. So although medication of the ADD person has its advantages, it's not always the panacea people expect it to be.

The important thing to remember about medication is that it is only one tool in the treatment process for people with ADD. The medical treatment of ADD really needs to be combined with a lot of other important tools for a successful relationship, tools like commitment, communication, conflict resolution skills, fun, and romance. Any one tool by itself will never be enough. Therapy can be a terrific place to pick up some tools people might have missed while growing up.

7) "If only we had kids—that would keep us together!"

Given the divorce rate in this country, and the well-publicized proliferation of single-parent families, it's hard to believe that people still cling to this particular myth. But for some reason, they do. "If we have a baby, then he'll have to become more responsible, more committed, more grounded." What kind of thinking is this? If the husband is already having those kinds of problems, more responsibility—when he can't handle what he's got already—is only going to make him bolt that much sooner. Or if he does stay, he still won't have the ability to access the part of his brain that makes things work better. Plus, there is a good possibility in this scenario that their biological offspring could have ADD and *really* challenge their lives. With a baby in the picture, the stress becomes too much for both of them to handle and the relationship blows apart.

It's mostly women who seem to buy into the idea of using a baby to try to make the other partner more responsible and committed. It's really just an extension of the Prince Charming concept. "After all, if he isn't my everything now, he'll have to become my everything when we have kids. I know he wouldn't leave me then. He wouldn't do that to me. And he certainly wouldn't do that to our little ones. If we could just have kids, he would never leave me. If we could just have kids, I know I would be secure."

Even sadder than the implications of this myth for the adult romantic relationship is what it means for the children. Because the subtext here is: "If my husband or partner doesn't meet my needs, these children surely will. If he won't become my everything, they will. If he leaves me, they never will. If he never loves me enough, I know the children will."

That's an awful burden to put upon a baby, isn't it? A healthy mother-child relationship involves the mother meeting the child's needs. That's the way it's supposed to work. Children aren't supposed to come into the world to meet their mother's needs. If you look at children as relationship problem-solvers, you haven't solved anything. All you've done is bring your own problems into yet another generation and increase the stress on an already overstressed relationship with your partner.

Of course, this isn't exclusively a women's issue. There are men who go through this, too. If they're insecure in their relationship with their wives, they might feel that a child will make their wife need them more—to help with child care if nothing else. Again, this is not an appropriate or optimistic foundation on which to build the relationship of your dreams.

Children bring a tremendous amount of joy to a family. But they also bring a significant amount of stress. In a family with a solid marital relationship, that stress can be managed appropriately. But if a married couple has significant problems, the stress of a child may worsen matters. It almost never makes things better.

Okay. We've gone over the seven most unrealistic expectations in a romantic relationship. Let's take a moment for a short review, and then we'll look at more realistic expectations to have about romantic relationships.

Unrealistic Expectations

1. All you need is love.
2. Now that we're married, everything should settle down and it will be smooth sailing from here on out.
3. I've meet the most wonderful guy. Finally. Someone who can meet all my needs.
4. I know she has problems. But she'll change if I just love her enough.
5. It's not my fault!
6. If he would just take his medication, everything would be fine.
7. If only we had kids—that would keep us together.

More Realistic Expectations for Romantic Relationships

1. Let's learn to live together. Learning how to love each other on a daily basis will sometimes be difficult— very difficult—but worth it.
2. The honeymoon phase is a lot of fun and important to our relationship. Let's enjoy it while it lasts, for soon the work of maintaining the relationship begins. As we learn our lessons well, we will be better able to

weather the storms of life which are sure to come our way.

3. No one but me is really responsible for my needs. I can enjoy what my partner brings to the relationship, but ultimately, it is my responsibility—not my partner's—to make certain my needs are met.

4. My partner and I are two separate individuals. I may need to change, but whether or not my partner needs to change is completely up to her. I accept and love my partner completely in this moment for who she is, not for who she might become.

5. In order for our relationship to work well, I must be willing to lay down my right to be right. There may be other, new possibilities I have never been able to see before because I have only looked at life through my eyes. The issue is not whose fault it was, but what I need to do differently in order for the two of us to grow and develop from the concept of "me" to the concept of "me and thee."

6. Whether or not my partner takes their ADD medication is ultimately their business. If invited to comment on their medication practices, I will do so. Otherwise that is their responsibility. My responsibility is to take care of my life and the responsibilities I have.

7. Our relationship will grow in positive ways if we work at learning and using new skills that will help us resolve conflict, communicate better, and have a mutually satisfying life together. If we can't get our act together without children, we'll never get it together with children.

Sounds like a lot of work . . . and it is. What makes it even scarier is that there's no guarantee that if you do all these things you will have the relationship of your dreams. Sorry, but that's the truth. But utilizing these more realistic expectations will ensure a more realistic view of what you are getting into—and help when the two of you encounter difficulties. Even though there's no guarantee, by applying these principles you have a much better chance of achieving a successful romantic relationship.

Discouraged? Don't be. This is what everyone faces with relationships . . . not just you. Do you feel like you need some tools to be better equipped for engineering a great relationship? Let's get started.

▼▲▼▲▼▲▼▲

FIVE

▲▼▲▼▲▼▲▼

ADD and the Challenges of Good Communication

So far, we've been hearing some frustrating and painful stories. Stories of ADD and romance that have been fairly discouraging, if not painfully familiar. That, my friend, is about to change. Up to this point we've had to paint a clear picture of ADD to better understand its damaging effects upon romantic relationships. Although we're still going to hear about people who have struggled in their relationships, let's shift our focus and look at concepts and tools you can use to make your relationship more loving, more connected, more gratifying, and more successful.

In any kind of relationship, good communication skills are a must. If you don't communicate well, the relationship won't last.

It doesn't matter whether we're talking about a father-son relationship, employer-employee, or a romantic relationship. In order to make the relationship work, in order for it to even have the chance to fulfill the expectations and needs of both parties to the best of their abilities, you have to talk *and* you have to listen.

It sounds so simple. But it rarely is.

We've all been involved in family problems in which one family member isn't really saying what they mean. Or maybe they're saying what they mean but constantly talking and never giving anyone else a chance to speak. We've all known of situations at work in which the boss says one thing—but really means something else. And far too many of us have been in romantic relationships that have fallen apart because the parties involved simply did not know how to sit down and communicate effectively with each other.

People can speak the same language to each other and still not understand the meaning of the communication. We each attach slightly different meanings to the words we use. That's a mechanical thing—later in this chapter we'll look at how to remedy that kind of problem. But there's yet another, more challenging problem in communicating with your partner. That's the challenge of sharing with them *who* you really are as a person, not just *what* you think . . . sharing your heart with them, the essence of your being.

Of course we already think we know how to do this. During the romancing phase of the relationship, we share our heart with our mate most of the time (or so we think). All those wonderful feelings of love. We write love letters and express ourselves clearly about our feelings—the fun feelings. We have long late-night phone conversations where we feel much but often speak very little. When we do speak, we hang onto each other's words.

But for people with ADD, building effective communication skills may be much more difficult than for the non-ADD population. Let's look at the symptoms of ADD that make good communication particularly difficult—impulsivity, difficulty staying on task, difficulty maintaining focus—and then discuss ways we can compensate for these symptoms to achieve more effective communication. But first, we need a strong foundation from which to build better communication skills.

Setting the Foundation for Good Communication

I want you to *really get* this next concept. It's the foundation we'll need for building better communication and maintaining a wonderful romantic relationship. Here it is: MOST CONFLICTS IN A ROMANTIC RELATIONSHIP ARE NOT ABOUT THE CON-FLICT — THEY ARE ABOUT SIGNIFICANCE.

Tattoo that sentence on your brain. Write it on your hand. Make sticky notes and put them on your bathroom mirror. Put them on the dash of your car. Put them anywhere you will see them. Memorize that sentence until it sinks into the deepest parts of your soul. Always place it in the forefront of your conscious thinking. That way, when you need it most, it will pop up and stare you in the face. It will act as a constant reminder of the direction you need to go in order to resolve conflicts and develop better communication skills so you can have the quality of relationship you deserve.

Significance. We all need it. We always have, beginning at birth. Without significance, babies die, from an affliction called "failure to thrive." "Failure to thrive" was identified at an orphanage where babies were having all of their basic physical needs met. They were sheltered from the elements, fed, clothed, and changed. If they had any medical needs, those needs were met by a full-time staff of doctors and nurses who were there around the clock to make certain they were healthy. Everything they needed physically was provided for. Still, babies died. It was baffling. By all rights, these babies should have flourished.

Then one day a nurse figured it out. She observed that the babies who were dying were those in the cribs against each of the four walls. These were the babies who were furthest away from human contact as the doctors and nurses walked through the ward. She also noticed that the babies who were thriving were the babies closest to the center aisle, and that as the doctors and nurses walked down that center aisle, they would always make eye contact with the babies and talk to them and touch them. Think about it. It's almost impossible to walk past an infant without being drawn to them in some way.

The babies who were doing well were the ones who experienced *significance*—the quality of feeling valuable, important, and loved—through the contact made by the doctors and nurses as they passed by. Since then, maternity wards have never been the same. Now you will find specific times set aside for mommy and baby to connect. You'll find rocking chairs and volunteer grandparents to rock and talk to the babies. When the baby's significance needs are being met (along with their other needs), the baby will thrive and flourish.

It's not that much different with us in romantic relationships. We don't need the eye contact an infant needs for developing a sense of significance, we're already adults. But, we definitely need to know and feel that we are significant to our partner—and vice versa—in order for the relationship to flourish. This sense of significance is so very important to each partner and to the well-being of the relationship.

Now, the reason I had you tattoo onto your brain that sentence—about conflicts being more about significance than they are about conflict—is because this concept plays a vital role in communication. When we listen to our partner and they listen carefully to us, here's the underlying message that comes across, no matter what the topic of conversation is: "You are significant to me. I want to know and understand you. I want to take the time to know who you really are. I want you to know that I care about you."

Good, clear communication is one of the tools we use to bond with each other and to have our significance needs met. We need to know that our voice is being heard, understood, and taken into consideration by our mate. Communication that does this is essential to the relationship. Believe it or not, having our significance needs met through good communication is often more important than getting our way or having our partner agree with us. Whether we're yelling at each other or whispering, both of us need to know and feel that we are significant enough to each other that our wants, needs, and desires are being heard. It doesn't mean we always get our way, but it does mean that our way merits equal consideration in the discussion. As I said earlier, most conflicts are not about the conflict, they are about significance. This will be a recurring theme through this chapter, so watch for it.

Common ADD Communication Behaviors

1) Not Talking

Sometimes people with ADD can talk too much. We'll take a look at that problem in a bit. But for now, we're going to take a look at not talking enough—especially about things that really need to be discussed with your partner.

It's possible that the ADD partner may not have a lot to say, or that they are too preoccupied with internal thought processes and forget to inform their partner as to what is going on inside of them. Possibly, they don't even know what they're supposed to talk about.

I remember when my own therapist told me years ago that I needed to communicate more with my wife. I didn't know what in the world he was talking about. I said, "I talk to my wife all of the time." I was certain he had to be mistaken. But the longer I stayed in therapy, the more I came to realize he was right.

There was a specific experience where the light bulb finally came on for me. My significant other was walking me to my gate at the airport. I was really struggling with financial problems at the time, and I was totally preoccupied with my internal thoughts and feelings and worries. I was definitely not fully present with her. All of a sudden my therapist's words about communicating more effectively came to me. I asked my companion, "By any chance are you aware that I am really scared right now about my personal financial situation?" She said, "No." I had been so caught up in my own internal worry/stimulation cycle that I hadn't clued her in on what was going on with me. My therapist had been right—I hadn't communicated very well.

We create intimacy by communicating with each other. But

when that communication is ineffective, intimacy flounders. I once heard someone say that they had a different spelling for intimacy: "into-me-see." Personally, that makes a lot of sense to me. It gets the point across that in order to be intimate, we need to let our partners see into the very essence of our being, see who we are in all of our splendor and all of our unsightliness. That can be frightening at times, but it doesn't have to be a big deal. In the example I was just talking about, it wasn't any secret that I was hurting financially. I just didn't know to share that with my significant other. Once I did, it helped her understand more of where I was coming from and who I was in that moment. Finally, I was starting to get what my therapist had been talking about. Communication in a romantic relationship is more than just talking. It is sharing your internal experiences—thoughts and emotions—with your partner.

If this is a problem you're familiar with, practice asking yourself every once in a while, "What am I thinking and feeling right now this very minute?" If it's a topic you and your mate have not talked about, or not talked about often, you might want to share what's going on inside of you with your partner. It may be valuable information for them to understand what you are going through and how that is affecting your behavior. It's also an opportunity for you to tell your partner that they are important enough to you to let them in on what you are going through. This kind of communication can help both of you grow closer together.

2) Impulsivity

This is a biggie for people with the hyperactive/impulsive component of ADD. They tend to speak their minds. That can be a very good thing. It's helpful to know where your partner really stands on issues, what their real thoughts and feelings are. However, there are times when we would all do better not to automatically speak our minds, and that's when poor impulse control tends to get people with ADD in trouble, over and over again. Yes, we'll speak our mind, but often at the wrong time—the proverbial "open mouth, insert foot" kind of speaking one's mind.

Stephen and Lila have been married for years. Stephen is the one with ADD, hyperactive/impulsive type, as you'll clearly see in just a moment. It's an extreme example, but I think you'll get the picture.

Stephen and his mother-in-law never really got along too well. They were cordial, but anyone who stayed around them enough could tell they were just being polite and tolerant of each other. Then Lila's mother died unexpectedly, early one morning in March. Stephen watched with great concern and compassion as Lila took the call from her dad that morning. He saw the tears flow down her face, and he held her as she cried in his arms when she got off the phone. So far, Stephen seems like a pretty good husband. But then he said in an attempt to comfort her, "She's probably happier where she is now." And as the next few words started to flow out of his mouth, he could feel in the pit of his stomach that what was about to take place was not going to be good. But it was too late. He said, "I know I am." Ouch. Let's run that back in slow motion to get the full impact of the sentence. "She's probably happier where she is now, I know I am."

How could he be so cruel? So insensitive? So thoughtless? So uncaring? The answer: ADD, hyperactive/impulsive type. Stephen would never have said anything like that to hurt his wife if he had the ability to edit his words before they came out of his mouth. He truly loves her and would never purposefully hurt her. It's more like he had the thought and the instant he had the thought is the same instant the words started rushing out of his mouth. He didn't realize how wrong it was until he said it, and by then he couldn't stop himself. In that micro-second before the words actually came out of his mouth, even he could sense that he was about to make a huge mistake.

It's been almost two years since that cold March morning in

Stephen and Lila's kitchen. Stephen has probably apologized a couple thousand times by now. He so wishes he could take the words back, but he can't. But with time, counseling and education about ADD, Stephen and Lila are both learning that decreased activity in the prefrontal cortex of Stephen's brain is often responsible for his impulsive words and actions.

Two years of pain brought on in less than two seconds because Stephen's brain was not able to operate fast enough to process what was about to come out. Had he the metabolic ability to consider the impact of his words before he spoke them, he never would have uttered them. He would have been able to edit himself.

Again, this is an extreme example of words spoken impulsively, but it does get the point across. Stephen has ADD, and even though he loves his wife, she was devastated by his impulsivity. Speaking his words at the exact moment he was thinking them caused a major breakdown in their communication, and in this particular instance, a major breakdown in their relationship.

The remedy? Medication would sure help make his prefrontal cortex work better, but there are also other things that can be done to help "control" the impulse. But it takes practice, practice, practice.

If you know you have impulse control problems with your speech, you need to develop a practice of reciting the next seven words in your head: BREATHE. THINK FIRST. THINK SLOWLY, THEN SPEAK. As I said before, this will take a lot of practice, but as we all know, practice makes perfect. Okay, for someone with ADD, not necessarily perfect, but moving in that direction.

The "BREATHE" part is very important for a lot of reasons. First, it slows down the communication process just a bit, which will help. Second, hyperactive people don't necessarily breathe well to begin with. When they become aroused—which is most of the time—they become shallow breathers. They just aren't getting enough oxygen into their system. They are in a somewhat altered state because their breathing is shallow. Learning deep breathing and practicing deep breathing can help to slow down the rapid-fire reflex of impulsive ADD speech.

The second part, words two and three, are "THINK FIRST." When you're saying this to yourself, you're further slowing down your response time. Remember, Stephen knew in his mind that the words coming out of his mouth were the wrong ones. He knew it as it was happening. Had he a second or two to slow the process down, he might have had the ability to mute the message before it was delivered. This second part of the counting is a self-command to consider what effect or outcome your message will have on your partner. It may be enough to hear this internal message, while slowing down the process, to develop some control.

Next is another internal self-directed message: "THINK SLOWLY." Here again, just repeating the words in your head slows the process down, adding precious micro-seconds to process information that is coming too fast to control in the first place. We are, through this practice, trying to put the brain into slow motion, or in the case of someone who has ADD, slow it down to a "normal" speed. Telling yourself not only to think about what is going on, but to think about it slowly, to consider as many angles, alternatives, and options as possible before you speak, slows the process down even more.

The last two words, "THEN SPEAK," give you permission to speak whatever it is you need to say. Will this work? Yes, it's possible for it to work, but it takes a lot of practice. Each of the steps is important. Will it always work? Probably not. Nothing is perfect. But if you're looking for tools to help control impulsivity, this is a good one. Here's a hint, though: It works a lot better with medication on-board.

Poor impulse control shows up in several communication problems. Another one of those problems is the ADHD tendency to interrupt the conversation—and even change the subject—when the other person is right in the middle of a sentence.

Let me give you an example that happened to me personally several years ago. I was on a trip with a friend of mine, driving in the country. Since she was doing the driving, I had the opportunity to just sit and enjoy the scenery, something I seldom get to do. My friend was talking to me about her new job and her concerns about her performance. I knew this was a very important subject to her. In fact, one of the reasons we had decided to take the drive in the first place was to discuss her feelings and concerns about her job.

"Excuse me just a moment, did you see that old car over there?" I asked excitedly.

"What?" She turned to look at me incredulously. "What are you talking about?"

"I'm talking about that old car over there. Back there in the field. Did you see it?"

The next thing I knew, my friend was angry at me. "Have you been listening to anything I've said?" she asked. "Anything at all? You know how difficult it is for me to talk in the first place, and then you don't even pay attention to me. That hurts! Now I don't even feel like talking to you at all!"

"Of course I was listening." Why was she acting so huffy all of a sudden, I wondered. After all, I didn't just butt in to her conversation. I used good manners. I was polite when I said "excuse me," wasn't I?

But to my friend, it was *exactly* like I just butted right into the conversation. Here she was talking about something very important to her. And she assumed, since I was someone who sincerely cared about her, that I would be able to recognize that importance. Instead, while she was divulging her deepest fears about her job to me, I interrupted to point out a car. Wow. I can certainly see how that would be painful and infuriating to her.

Often, the person with ADD will interrupt the communication from their partner by saying, "Excuse me, I don't mean to change the subject, but . . ." and then abruptly change the subject entirely.

To the ADD partner, that request seems perfectly valid. It's not that they're trying to be rude, even though it certainly feels that way to the other partner. What's really happening at that very moment is the interrupting partner all of a sudden gets a thought in their mind. They feel a tremendous amount of internal pressure to get this particular thought out into the conversation. So they butt in, albeit "politely." They sometimes assume that if they ask politely enough, their partner won't have any trouble with it. Wrong. This kind of behavior is very disconcerting.

Now we're getting somewhere. Instead of thinking the interrupter is an inconsiderate oaf, we're wondering why in the world they did that. What's taking place in the mind of the ADD person that they would act in such a way? Here's the answer.

People with hyperactive/impulsive ADD have a brain that races a thousand miles a minute. It's constantly rushing from one idea to the next. It's one of the plusses and drawbacks of having ADD. In conversation, if something is said that sparks another—seemingly unrelated—thought in their mind, *that* thought will catch their attention. But because they know their mind rushes so fast, they also know that new thought may only stay in their mind for a split second. They believe it's important information to give to you even though they know it's totally unrelated to what you might be talking about. Fearful that this important thought might be lost forever in the ever-rushing flood of other thoughts, they blurt out, as politely as they know how in the intensity of that moment, "Excuse me, I don't mean to change the subject, but . . ." And they're off and running. They're afraid that if they don't say it in that instant, they'll forget it.

All of this makes sense as to why there is such intensity to their impulsive interruptions. But when we interrupt and change subjects in that way, it sabotages the other person's sense of significance. No matter how polite we try to be, the message we send to our partner—when we interrupt and change the subject—is that they really aren't important to us. Our message supersedes their message—and their feelings. We are indicating that what we have to say is much more important than what they have to say. And that is terribly demeaning and hurtful to our partner. That definitely sabotages their sense of significance and attacks their innate value.

When a non-ADD person has an ADD partner (or when both are ADD but one is a little more ADD than the other), both partners need to work at understanding these kinds of situations. The ADD partner needs to try to understand how demeaning these impulsive interruptions feel to his or her partner. And the non-ADD partner needs to understand that these interruptions are not about behavior that is purposefully demeaning. These impulsive interruptions aren't even about the relationship between the two people at all. The impulsiveness, as frustrating as it is, is only about ADD. Period.

For the non-ADD partner, the interruption, the urgency behind the interruption may be difficult to understand. After all, if you don't have ADD, you can usually control your impulses. You learned as a child how to do that. The ADD person tried as hard as they could as a child to learn that, but it didn't work because their brain doesn't give them that ability. But imagine that *you* were a "prisoner of the moment," so to speak, and you had something really important to say. Now imagine that you're not allowed to communicate that to your partner—at all. Wouldn't that feel unfair? Wouldn't you feel left out? When the ADD partner is forced to wait—and, in their mind, wait and wait and wait—to make their point, *they* feel like *their* significance has been diminished. Because they feel that if they cannot get their "stuff" heard, then *their* "stuff" is insignificant. Ergo, *they* are insignificant. That's why it is so important to partners (and therapists, and doctors, and teachers, etc.) to know what is ADD behavior and what is not. When we know what ADD behaviors look like and how they affect romance, we are better able to *not* take things so personally.

No one really likes being seen as rude and self-centered. Like Stephen, whom we talked about earlier in this section, the impulsivity happens at the same time the brain is thinking—sometimes before the individual even knows *what* they are thinking. It is very frustrating for both partners.

One easy-to-understand method to short-circuit this urge is for the ADD person to carry a notebook and pencil around with them. If they have an instantaneous thought they want to get across while their partner is talking, they can write it down—just a word or two that will remind them—so that when it is their turn, they can then share that thought without fear that it will be lost. Of course, people with ADD often lose pencils and notebooks quicker than you can imagine. This tool may work for some people—it's worth a try. But don't be discouraged or disheartened if it doesn't. This may be one of those things that both of you need to learn to accept as part of the territory.

Being gentle with each other at this point can help a lot. "She's just being real ADD right now. I love her with all of my heart. Yes, this is frustrating, but it's not about me, or about us. It's not about anything other than her ADD." Often this acceptance approach is the best because it deals with reality instead of fantasy (of changing the impulsive behavior). Choose your battles. Learn how to decide what is really important to you and what you can let go of. That will help both of you as a couple and as individuals.

One way people with ADD try to show their partners that they're paying attention is by finishing their sentences for them. They have the best of intentions, but if you've ever been in a conversation like that, you know how frustrating it can be. It often goes something like this:

Norm is trying to tell Helen about the meeting he had earlier that day with his mother's doctor. Helen, who has ADD, is paying close attention. She cares about Norm's mother and wants him to know how genuinely concerned she is.

"I had a great meeting with Mom's doctor this morning," he says. "He took the time to—"

"—Show you all her test results?"

"No. He took the time to explain each of her medications. He told me which ones—"

"—Which ones she had to take with food and which ones on an empty stomach?"

"No. He told me which ones she has to take in the morning and which ones she has to take at night. But the most important thing was that he warned me to watch her very carefully—"

"—To see if she develops a fever. I know you have to watch for infection."

"No. He warned me to watch carefully and make sure—"

"—That the medications don't make her dizzy. I know that can happen when you're taking too many medications. You know when my dad was sick last year he had that problem, too. He had . . ."

"You know what? That isn't what I was going to say at all. But just forget it. Just forget the whole thing," Norm says.

"What did I do? I was trying to pay close attention to what you were saying," Helen says, and she is genuinely confused. But by this time Norm is exhausted, frustrated, and disgruntled from the effort of trying to complete any sentence before Helen cuts him off. Is this a good thing? No. Is it ADD-type behavior? Absolutely. Is the ADD affecting the ability of the couple to communicate effectively? Definitely.

One of the tools I teach couples to use when in this kind of situation is called "the talking stick." The talking stick is a tool for effective communication that Native Americans have used to make certain everyone gets their say in a matter. The talking stick and the person holding it are allowed to speak their mind without interruption. It's a very effective tool for helping couples to direct verbal traffic and reduce the incidence of mid-sentence collisions. You can use anything you want as a talking stick. A pencil. A spoon. You could even use a watermelon if you wanted to. Passing that big thing back and forth (not throwing!) could really slow down the communication process, and the impulsivity as well. The idea I teach in counseling is that whoever holds the talking stick has control of the conversation. The listener is not to interrupt. They are to listen. When the speaker is done, they relinquish the talking stick to their partner. Then *they* have the full attention of the other person. The partners pass it back and forth, equally sharing their ideas, their feelings, their thoughts until they have each had their say. Once all of the information is out on the table, they can begin to problem-solve. But not before then. It's a great tool. I also use it with families in which the whole family impulsively interrupts each other. It works wonderfully.

There are some pitfalls to watch out for in this process, such as not listening when you don't have the talking stick. All too often, we don't listen to our partner when they're talking—even though we're not interrupting—because we're too busy planning our rebuttal. We get caught up in "my way" thinking instead of approaching the problem with a mind-set of "let's see what we can come up with *together* so that both of us get what we want." Relationships run a lot smoother when each partner makes sure that they both get their needs met and work together as a team instead of against each other.

3) Subject Changing

Here's one a lot of us go through, though we may not know it's even happening. Have your ever had a conversation with someone who, throughout the conversation, continually changed the subject you were trying to discuss? Maddening, isn't it? All you get is emotionally exhausted and frustrated. There is never any resolution to the issue at hand. And no one's significance needs ever get met.

Conversations that change directions as often as the ADD person has a new thought in their mind can be very frustrating.

This particular communication dilemma is one of the most serious problems caused by ADD in romantic relationships, and probably a major contributor to the demise of many relationships. Why? Nothing ever gets resolved. Besides the different kinds of problems we have already discussed, there are the ongoing frustrations of never getting the original problems resolved. Those frustrations may then take a deadly toll on the relationship. At that point the relationship, which may have seemed like the *Love Boat* at first, ends up feeling more like the *Titanic*. When the couple's unsinkable love for each other hits an iceberg in a sea full of unresolved conflicts, all that's left to discuss is who will go down with the ship. Before *that* solution is ever found, the conversation takes on seventeen new directions and before you know it, both partners are watching fish through their cabin porthole while the band plays on.

One of the problems I see so often when I'm working with couples in which ADD is present is that the subject of a conversation gets changed constantly. And it's usually not even because the ADD person is purposefully trying to change the subject. But it makes it next to impossible to resolve any conflict because they don't have the skills to stay on task with any one subject long enough to resolve it.

Here's the way it usually happens: The first person makes a comment about something—let's say, a particular behavior in their partner that they don't like. When the ADD partner hears that comment, it triggers something in his mind that is closely related, but in a different direction. He begins talking about that new topic. It's a closely related topic, so she follows his lead in that direction. Once or twice more and suddenly, the couple is arguing about a totally different topic. At the end of their conversation, both partners feel battered and exhausted. The topic of conversation changed so many times that neither partner felt heard, neither partner felt significant, and neither partner knows how in the world they ever got from point A to point Z.

What I do with clients who converse like this is first help them to become aware of what they are doing. Often they deny that they constantly change the direction of the conversation. I may simply point it out. I may, with their consent, videotape them in one of these multi-directional conflicts and then play the tape back so they can see for themselves what was taking place. After all, a picture is worth a thousand denials.

Then it's just a mechanical solution. I teach the couple to write down the main point of what they want to get across, and the couple then dialogues, utilizing paraphrasing, until the message sent is the same as the message received. We use paraphrasing—not parroting—because it gives the sender of the communication a clear picture of the message received. The original root word *para* is Greek, and means "alongside of." A paraphrase is a phrase that is alongside the original phrase. Paraphrasing means not repeating the exact same words that the original sender used. That would be parroting. Parroting is not beneficial because it is possible to repeat the same words without really understanding the meaning of their message. Paraphrasing, on the other hand, allows the sender to know whether or not they were really understood. Then I teach the couple to stay focused on one issue—using the tool of paraphrasing—until that specific issue is resolved. Once that issue is resolved, then they can move on to the next issue.

Both partners are advised to be on the watch for abrupt changes. If that happens, they should identify there has been a change (tangent), circumnavigate the change, and stay on course by finding resolution to that specific issue before they move on to anything else.

This is nothing more than structure. And although structure can often be difficult for people with ADD to embrace, it's much easier when they can see the need for structure (via videotape feedback) on their own, and then choose to add this structure to their communication process as a way to help them keep their own, personal love boat afloat.

4) Low Self-esteem

When a person has been told year after year and decade after decade that they're not good enough—that they make stupid mistakes, that they mess up time and time again, that they're an "airhead" (or some other demeaning label)—it's not surprising they have low self-esteem. Those feelings of low self-esteem can manifest themselves in communication problems as well as in many other ways. Because of this, people with ADD can easily develop communication patterns of being on the defensive almost all of the time, in almost every conversation. And when you feel like you always have to be on the defensive—whether, in fact, anyone is accusing you of anything or not—you spend an awful lot of time and energy developing your case, so to speak. And not nearly enough time really listening to what your partner is saying.

This conversation is very similar to the type we just talked about, where the ADD person changes the subject umpteen million times and nothing gets resolved. Except this time the response is a defense of some kind, or worse yet, an attack. After all, the best defense is a good offense (or so we may mistakenly believe).

Here's an example: Ken and April have been dating for a brief period of time when Ken mentions to April that he would like for her to call him sometimes, rather than just him calling her. April hears this not as an invitation but as a criticism—as if she isn't doing something the right way . . . again. Her response is in no way rude, but it does catch Ken by surprise. "I would have started calling you a long time ago if I knew you wanted me to." Notice she isn't directly saying that she would love to call him, even though she really would love to call him. Instead, she places the responsibility for her "inaction" back on him. A gentle yet defensive response. A subtle form of "it wasn't my fault"—a common phrase in the vocabulary of just about every ADD person. When they know each other better, it may become much less subtle. Ken says to April at the end of a wonderful evening together, "I wish we could have had more time together tonight." She responds, "It wasn't my fault. I got stuck in traffic and the dry cleaners closed before I could get my dress out for tonight, so I had to rush to the store and find a new one!" Then, after they're married, April takes the "best offense" approach. When Ken says, "You know, honey, I'd sure like it if when you finish off a roll of toilet paper that you'd put a new one in the dispenser." She replies, "Well, you never do!" At that point her defense turns into an attack.

Defend. Defend. Defend. Understandably, after a lifetime of feeling criticized and ridiculed, these kinds of responses will show up. Therapy can be helpful for this. Even if you get this person on the right medication for their brain, the wounds to their self-esteem are still there. Therapists are often able to help people with these kinds of issues. Plus, the more the ADD person feels "safe" with their partner, the more they can learn to trust them and let down their guard. And the more they will realize they don't have to be hyper-vigilant, ready to defend their ego at the drop of a hat as they've had to do so many times before.

5) Pressured Speech

Have you ever known anyone with ADD, particularly the hyperactive type of ADD, who talked all the time? The rapid-fire kind of talk where you wonder if they will ever take a breath? If you've ever been in a romantic relationship with someone like that, you probably thought you'd never get a word in edgewise.

Some people who have the hyperactive type of ADD feel a tremendous need to get all their information out there, all at once. They have a constant underlying fear that they'll forget something. And because they're so hyperfocused on their own issues and the points they feel an intense need to make in a conversation, they are often unaware of their partner's needs or desires at that time. One thought runs into the next, and there's no time to take a breath to shift attention to their partner. At that point the communication really changes from a conversation to a monologue. The ADD person is talking and talking and talking, and oblivious to the fact that their partner would like to participate in the conversation too. This can and will certainly sabotage significance needs if left untreated. Medical interventions could help tremendously, as would education for both partners about ADD and how it is affecting their relationship. At least then they can blame the cause and not the victims of the cause.

A contributor to this particular communication problem is the person with ADD thinking out loud. That is, they need to speak what they are thinking and hear their thoughts with their own ears in order to really understand what they're thinking. It's almost like hearing yourself talk and figuring out the issue at the same time. This is not the case for everyone who has ADD. Literally, the ADD person is processing that information externally the way most people process information internally. This is not the case for everyone who has ADD, but it is an ADD processing problem that happens for a lot of people.

Usually, pressured speech is really more about a need for stimulation combined with a fear that they will leave out something important. These communication problems are yet additional indicators of the need for medication. Helping the individual slow down the communication process by identifying that they are "running" with their communication can be very beneficial for them when done gently and lovingly But you've got to remember, that rapid-fire pace—their pressured speech—is also serving a purpose: self-stimulation.

Here's a brief story about how significant that stimulation can be for someone. A patient I was working with in the hospital had pressured speech. The more he talked in group therapy with his rapid-fire, run-on sentences, the more the rest of the group became angry, unable to get a word in edgewise.

One day I turned to Nigel and gently pointed out that he was talking very fast and asked him to slow down. He worked and worked at it. He would slow down, then stop for just a second, then take off talking again. Finally, after lots of gentle coaching, he was able to sit still and not say a word. At that moment he began to weep openly. He felt so uncomfortable in his own body because his brain wasn't working right that he just couldn't stand it. His speech was pressured because he was both self-stimulating and self-medicating his internal sense of "dis-ease" through the distraction of nonstop talking.

There are medications that can help people like Nigel feel better and function better by helping their brains work the way they're supposed to work. That's why I say that people with this particular symptom of ADD would probably function a lot better in life and love relationships with the aid of medication.

6) Not Remaining Focused

William is in his thirties and in his second marriage. As he looks back on his first marriage, he believes it failed due to one particular communication problem caused by his then-undiagnosed ADD: He could not really be present with his wife even when she was talking to him and looking into his eyes. His mind was in far-off places, daydreaming about who knows what. William didn't know any different. He was being the way he had always been. And he could track most of what she was saying. But still, she saw that far-off, distant look in his eyes—a look she mistook for his not caring about her enough to really focus on her. This was excruciatingly painful for her. He was a good man. He never cheated on her. But still, she felt alone even when she was with him. Eventually they separated and divorced.

It's so sad that every year thousands of marriages break up over this kind of experience. When she told William she wasn't sure if she really wanted to be married to him anymore, it really took him by surprise. "What did I do?" he would ask, over and over. All she could say was, "I just don't feel you love me." And William would answer, "I couldn't love anyone more than I love you." They both hurt unbelievably. They would both tell you that they still loved each other. But William's wife just couldn't take the loneliness anymore. It's a sad but common story for people involved with someone who has ADD.

A few years later, after many of the wounds and scars had healed and William had recovered from the divorce, he met someone new whom he could love. Someone he was willing to trust again for love and companionship. After years of therapy, his psychiatrist diagnosed him as having ADD and put him on medications. William was still the same guy, but now his brain could process things better. Now he could be more present with people.

Sandra was the new woman in his life. She was vivacious. Caring. Nurturing. Successful. Wonderful. They met at a support group for adults at their church. Both had been married before. Both had similar kinds of experiences, so they had that common ground to bond on, along with all of the other things they enjoyed about each other. William suspected that Sandra might also have ADD. He was just learning about it himself, but wondered if she might also have difficulty staying on task, like him. He brought it up in conversation. She suggested he was just seeing that in her because he was so excited about the changes he was seeing in himself as a result of the medication he was taking. He was willing to consider that, although some of the symptoms his doctor had identified in him also seemed present in her too.

Then one day it happened, long after the honeymoon phase was over. Now that he was on a therapeutic dose of neurostimulant—now that the endorphin rush was over and things were settling down in the relationship—he got to experience what his first wife had complained of but didn't understand.

On this particular day William had just secured a huge contract with a company he had been courting for some time. His hard work and diligence had finally paid off. This contract would ensure them a steady and sizable income for years to come. They could now relax a little and take that special honeymoon they had talked about but couldn't afford the time off to take.

William rushed home to tell Sandra the great news. As he was sharing with her what had happened, she smiled and nodded in all of the right places, but she didn't really seem to be present with him. Sure she liked the idea of finally being able to go on the special honeymoon and relax a bit more, but still she didn't seem to care. She didn't share that same electricity William was experiencing. After a few minutes of this, William lost a lot of his enthusiasm. Feeling confused and hurt, he turned and walked away to the den by himself.

William stayed alone in the den for a while that evening. He wasn't angry, he felt hurt and alone. He knew Sandra loved him, but something wasn't right. Then he got it. He finally understood. Sandra had just given him a wonderful gift to help him let go of the painful question that had haunted him these last few years in spite of all his therapy.

William finally understood what his first wife was talking about when she left him, even though she loved him so much. She hurt the way William was hurting that very moment. He cried tears of relief and tears of pain for his first wife. Had he known back then what Sandra had just revealed to him this night, they might never have gotten divorced. He ached for the pain she had gone through all those years, day after day, when she would talk intimately about her day and he could only be partly present in the conversation. How she had suffered! Now he knew.

When it comes to communication in intimate relationships, our partner needs us to be 100 percent attentive to them in order for them to experience the significant place they hold in our heart. Without that ongoing sense of significance for both partners, the relationship will falter and most likely die.

If you already take medication for your ADD, make certain it is "on-board" in your body when you and your mate are talking intimately. Make certain you have done everything you know to guarantee that when you and your mate are communicating, you are both fully present. Turn the TV off so you can't be distracted by that. Send the kids to bed, or wait until they are asleep. Then connect and communicate, able to be fully present without distraction. If it's just a quick moment for a brief message, turn away from the computer screen so that while your beloved is speaking to you they have your undivided attention. Do everything you can to be fully present with them, emotionally, spiritually, and mentally. This is very important.

It has been estimated that nearly ten percent of the entire population has ADD and that only two percent of all those people have been diagnosed and treated for their ADD. Millions of people are experiencing the kind of "alone-ness" and pain we just described above. What about you? If, after reading this material, you think you might have ADD, do something about it. Find a professional who knows ADD inside and out and get the help both you and your partner need and deserve. Don't let your undiagnosed and untreated ADD be the unknown root cause of pain in your relationship.

Likewise, if you are experiencing what we have been talking about and you don't have ADD but are involved with someone who does, learn all you can about ADD. Educate yourself so you can identify what is and is not ADD behavior. That way you can make better decisions for your life in terms of relationship challenges.

7) Obsessive Thinking

Let's throw yet another monkey wrench into the works. When a person has an overactive cingulate gyrus (the brain system discussed in Chapter Two) in addition to the prefrontal cortex problems that result in ADD symptoms, they will also tend to get stuck in their thinking to the exclusion of almost everything else. Once they lock onto an idea, they can't let it go.

Such was the case for Mel and Tanya. This was one of those "on again/off again" kinds of relationships. Real intense. Real stimulating.

During one of their "off again" moments, after they had been apart for nearly nine months, Mel took a female colleague to lunch one afternoon. It was only a lunch. No hanky-panky. No nothing. Just lunch. Besides, he was a single man again. He and Tanya hadn't dated in nine months. But that weekend, Tanya contacted Mel and told him how much she missed him and how much she wanted to be with him again, that her life was miserable without him.

Taking the bait, Mel jumped right back into the relationship with Tanya, right where they left off.

While Mel and Tanya were watching TV together that Sunday night, Mel's colleague from the office called to see if she could return the favor and take him to lunch on Monday. Mel, feeling rather awkward, declined. He told his co-worker that he and Tanya were back together again and he was now unavailable.

Tanya was outraged. Another woman calling him! Pursuing her man! How could he treat her so thoughtlessly? She jumped up from the couch, grabbed her jacket, and stormed out the door. They talked on the phone late that night, and many nights for months after that. Just about when things were starting to get better between them, she would bring up the lunch date. Over and over and over again. Mel would always say, "But we weren't together then! You broke up with me, and I had seen no one for nine months. What was I supposed to do? Join a monastery for the rest of my life?"

Whenever there was an argument—or when things just got too quiet in the relationship—Tanya would bring up the lunch date.

Mel felt so frustrated, as if he were on the hook for something he did wrong when he hadn't done anything wrong. And there was never any forgiveness from Tanya. She just couldn't let go of "the lunch date." Mel was emotionally bludgeoned for this "thoughtless act" time and time again.

Want to hear something that is really amazing? Tanya would say that she understood they were not a couple when it happened and that he had been totally free to see whomever he wanted—and in the same breath tell him again that she just couldn't get over how thoughtless he had been. How callous he was to have hurt her like that. The thought was stuck in her mind, and she kept saying the same thing over and over again.

Both Mel and Tanya have ADD. Different types of ADD, but nonetheless, both have ADD. The communication between the two of them fails—as does their relationship—for several reasons. First of all, neither is on medication for their ADD. Their communication falters because they are using the intensity—both positive and negative intensity—to stimulate their brains. Their ongoing communication pattern serves to stimulate them rather than draw them closer together. Their communication is not about intimacy, it's about stimulation. That's the first reason they struggle with communication. But the second reason is Tanya's overactive cingulate gyrus. She just can't let go. Her obsessiveness feeds the stimulation she derives from communicating with Mel. But they can't stop. In essence, since they're both using each other for stimulation—for the drug they want to make their brains feel better—they're very much addicted to each other . . . not in love with each other. What can they do?

What could salvage this relationship, if there really is a relationship here, is medication. They both need to have their prefrontal cortex activated so they can think more clearly and understand that this is a very sorry relationship. Tanya needs additional medication for her "stuck" cingulate. When, through pharmacological interventions, her cingulate calms down some and gives her the ability to shift better, that will also help their relationship.

How about counseling? There are some psychotherapeutic interventions that have shown promise for treating overactive cingulates. But before Tanya can get any help for her cingulate, she will first need to admit she gets stuck in her thinking, and the chance of that happening is slim, because Tanya is stuck on the idea that she's not the one with the problem. Either way, this couple is destined to be miserable until they get the metabolic functioning of their brains under control—and get into counseling or therapy to learn more positive and productive communication skills.

8) Not Receiving the Intended Message

It's not uncommon for people with ADD to also have problems in the temporal lobe region of the brain. The temporal lobes are located in the area behind your temples on both the left and right sides of your brain. Anomalies in the functioning of the temporal lobes can also cause communication problems. Because these problems are a result of brain system dysfunction, it's best to think of them as being "mechanical" problems instead of problems of will. These mechanical problems can make it difficult for the person to physically hear correctly and interpret and understand language. Often, people with this type of problem will misinterpret comments as being negative, when they're actually not negative comments at all. They feel attacked, even though their partner is not attacking them. And they feel that way because they're not able to understand the comments correctly. Their ears may work fine, but their brain, because of a "mechanical" malfunction, switches it all around and things are heard with a negative spin on them. This mechanical problem most often has to do with temporal lobe dysfunction.

For example, Jane is a woman with ADD who has a coexisting

language problem related to problems in her left temporal lobe. She experiences the symptoms I just described. A few months ago, her car wouldn't work right and needed to be taken into the shop. So she asked her boyfriend, Brian, if he could take her to work the following morning. Brian is a nighttime kind of guy—definitely not a morning person. But Jane had to be at work at 7 a.m., and she has an hour commute to work. Did Brian really want to do this? Yes. But having to get up at 5 a.m. was a big push for him. Still he sincerely wanted to help Jane out. So he set his alarm, miraculously woke up, and was at Jane's apartment at 5:45 a.m.

"You know what this means, don't you?" he asked Jane as they walked to his car from her apartment. "For me to be up this early to take you to work means I really, really love you." And he meant it.

But Jane, because of her temporal lobe dysfunction, was horribly offended at Brian's comment. Since she has ADD she also has little impulse control, the ability to think things through first. *"What did you mean by that?"* she asked, practically screaming at him—and fully ready to walk to work instead of ride with Brian.

Brian, of course, was at a loss. He had gotten up very early, which was difficult for him to do, and then when he tried to explain to Jane how much love was behind his actions . . . she became enraged. The problem is that Jane, because of her ADD and temporal lobe dysfunction, was physically unable to correctly interpret what Brian was actually saying. That part of her brain (her temporal lobe) that processes a lot of communication information wasn't working right and put a negative spin on the way she heard what Brian had said. She understood something different from what Brian had said, jumped to conclusions, and all but scratched his eyes out when he was trying to tell her how much he loved her.

ADD and temporal lobe dysfunction, when combined with Jane's problem of getting stuck in her thinking, can lead to some very bad possibilities. In our research at The Amen Clinic, we have found that this particular combination of anomalies in the brain—

decreased activity of the prefrontal cortex (ADD), overactive cingulate (obsessive), and both increased and decreased activity of the temporal lobes (anger, auditory processing problems, misinterpretation of comments)—often leads to domestic violence. We'll get back into straight ADD in just a second but first, I want you to know that if you are in a situation in which you are fearful of the possibility of domestic violence, see a therapist. There are a lot of factors involved in domestic violence, including brain metabolism. But don't become a victim. If there's a problem and you really love this person, it may still work out, but you both will need counseling to prevent domestic violence. If you're already in such a relationship and violence is taking place, call the local hotline for battered women in your community, call the police, or call a therapist or physician and ask for help. It's up to you to stay safe. You can always work on having the relationship of a lifetime *after* the two of you get those things handled.

9) Brain Melt-Down

When a person with ADD is in conflict, he can react in one of two ways. He can either become totally stressed, in which case his prefrontal cortex can shut down completely, or he can be stimulated by the conflict and seek to prolong it as much as possible. Either way, his communication capabilities and consequently his partner also suffer.

Through our use of SPECT brain imaging—which uses nuclear medicine to take pictures of brain activity—we have seen over and over again that when people with ADD are under a lot of stress, their prefrontal cortex shuts down. That's the reason kids with ADD have such a difficult time performing well on the traditional types of tests given in school—they have brain melt-down. And that's the reason communication often shuts down when the ADD partner senses, whether correctly or not, that he is coming under attack from his partner. When the prefrontal cortex shuts down, the ADD partner finds it very difficult to sort through his thoughts, much less take in yet more information from his partner. And chances are he might just withdraw into himself and stop communicating altogether with his partner.

This is, of course, frustrating for the partner. After all, the partner might want to resolve the conflict through continued communication. Instead, the ADD partner just seems to shut down. He might turn away from his partner—or even walk out of the room. In reality, the partner with ADD might need communication, and the bonding that it brings, more than ever. But he can't access that if his prefrontal cortex shuts down. Unless you're both aware of significance needs like we talked about in the first part of this chapter, someone's feelings are going to get hurt.

When the ADD person experiences brain melt-down, they have difficulty processing information. They may feel a bit confused and have difficulty identifying what they are feeling, both emotionally and physically. The best thing to do is give them some space, physically and emotionally, to gather their thoughts and regroup. A few slow, deep breaths would help them to relax a bit and allow their brain to return to a higher level of functioning.

10) Conflict-Seeking Behavior

As we've discussed in an earlier chapter, many people with ADD find conflict to be incredibly stimulating. And that stimulation makes them feel better. So they seek that stimulation through conflict whenever possible—although they probably don't realize what they're doing. In this case, real and meaningful communication becomes almost impossible. How can you really communicate with someone who is doing everything they possibly can to get you to fight with them?

In addition the ADD partner may become even more verbal

than normal because of the stimulation brought on by the conflict. And he might have more difficulty than normal with impulse control, saying things now he will regret later.

All in all, it's a real recipe for disaster: conflict-seeking, impulsive, over-the-top communication. Not exactly the kind of stuff that makes for great relationships.

That's exactly what was happening with one couple I worked with. No matter what Edgar did or didn't do, or what he did or didn't say, his wife, Diane, was always angry with him.

Finally, one day, Edgar had had enough. He had let himself be pushed into one too many fights. He became very quiet and turned to Diane and said, "You know, I think I could hear you better if you weren't screaming so much."

And that's when Diane turned to him and said, "I like to be angry. I feel good when I'm angry!"

That one tiny conversation summed up so much about their relationship. Because Diane had ADD, she felt better in her own body when she was self-medicating with adrenaline—adrenaline she self-generated through angry, conflict-seeking behaviors. That was good for her. But it definitely wasn't good for Edgar. And it wasn't good for their relationship.

If you see these kinds of things happening in *your* relationship, I hope you can take notice of them and identify the ADD characteristics we're talking about. Then follow the steps that Edgar and Diane took to find better ways to connect and communicate. Find a professional who really knows ADD inside and out, and get some treatment. Diane's physician prescribed medication to treat her ADD. Through counseling, Edgar and Diane have been able to learn more appropriate and productive communication skills. Diane learned that she developed a habit of self-stimulating through conflict and decided she wanted to break that habit. The medication helps Diane tremendously in understanding her behaviors and also in diminishing her need to seek stimulation through conflict. Now when Diane begins to seek conflict, she can catch herself and choose to interact more appropriately. Through this process, she is consciously choosing to change. Edgar and Diane are now beginning to enjoy their relationship and each other. Their hard work in therapy and the benefits of medication are helping them become a much happier couple.

Negotiating Resolution

Conflict resolution is difficult for a lot of couples. A lack of adequate conflict resolution skills can really bog down a relationship. I want to share with you a quick and easy-to-understand approach for resolving conflict. Easy to understand, but not necessarily easy to apply. Here's how it works.

First and foremost, remember something you learned earlier in this chapter—the importance of making sure you and your partner's significance needs are being met. Most conflicts are more about significance than they are about the conflict. So the first place you look for resolution is by figuring out whether or not significance is the real issue. If it is, then talk about feeling insignificant to your partner. Talk about your pain. Be vulnerable and share what hurts you. Do this without attacking them. If they become defensive, reassure them that you are not out to hurt them, you just want them to understand your feelings.

When my wife and I practice this, she will verbally remind herself that this is not about having to do something she doesn't want to do. It is not about having to take care of me or even do what I want. It's about listening to me and letting me know she understands what I'm feeling and why I'm feeling that way. Then, if *she* wants to, she can do something about it or do absolutely nothing about it. That's totally up to her. My job is not to coerce her into doing what I want. That wouldn't be love. That would be manipulation. Manipulation is not love. Love is a free choice. My job is to present to her as clearly and concisely as possible what I feel, what I want, what I need. Period.

When couples practice this approach, it makes it much easier to resolve conflict because no one is having to give up something they don't want to. Whatever they give is a gift because it's of their own free will.

Once the significance needs are addressed and there is still a conflict, the next step is to form a partnership—after all, that's what you're supposed to be anyway, isn't it? The following is your goal as partners in negotiating resolution: Do everything in your power to make certain your partner's wants and needs are being met to the same degree that you are working to make certain your own wants and needs are being met. When you are both striving toward that goal, your partner doesn't have to fight with you any longer. They know you're pulling for what they want too.

When you achieve this mind-set, you can put the real conflict out on the negotiating table and work as a team to make certain that both of you get what you want. This can be a rewarding exercise for some ADD people because they can be very creative. This is a creative process. Couples usually find that when they follow these "simple" precepts they can use real conflict to create real intimacy. Not only are they able to problem-solve better, but when they have successfully negotiated a resolution, they have actually strengthened their relationship through the process and can celebrate their joint success. It may take some practice, but if the two of you can do this, it will revolutionize your relationship.

Not all conflicts can be resolved this way. There might be times when both of you are at such opposite extremes that you won't be able to find one solution that works for both of you. What to do then? Ever hear of the old cliche "agree to disagree"? It's a cliche for a reason. But when both of you have your significance needs being met, it's a lot easier to let go and allow yourselves the room to agree to disagree. Then do what you need to do as individuals. It's so much easier to do this when you have developed a deeper sense of intimacy by struggling through the processes we just talked about.

How to Improve Communication with an ADD Partner

Here's a great tool to learn how to listen better and communicate more clearly. It's called Emotional Mapping. Emotional Mapping takes time to learn, which means you'll both need to practice it. In time, if you learn how to use this tool effectively, your communication will improve without even having to adhere to the rigid template for communication I'm about to give you. But don't be in too big a hurry to get there. It's like training wheels on a bicycle. You both need to use your training wheels until you have enough self-confidence to ride on your own. Besides, even after all of your practice, you can easily fall back onto the structure in times of conflict when you need a bit more structure to succeed. At first, when learning this process, it may take some time to get through the whole thing, so plan at least a half hour to an hour. Also, both of you need to agree in advance on a practice time.

First, face each other and hold hands. The first person, "the sender," says, "What I'm angry about is . . ." and then fill in that blank with *brief*, factual information. For example, "What I'm angry about is that you didn't show up at 5 p.m. today to pick me up like you had said you would." It's not appropriate to say something like, "What I'm angry about is you're such an inconsiderate jerk." That's not factual information. It may be what you'd like to say out of your anger, but it's not the best way to communicate. "Jerk" could be debated every which way to Sunday because it is not factual, and besides that, it is a derogatory term that is certain to offend your mate. Time. Date. Place. Specific facts. And it needs to be brief. If the sentences get too long, as in paragraphs, it's probably too much information for your partner to take in. You'll need to keep it brief and concise because in a moment, your partner is going to have to paraphrase it back to you. Go easy on them. Make it short.

Next, "the receiver" paraphrases back what the sender said. Don't "parrot" it back—don't use the same words. You don't want to echo them. If you did that, it might only signify that you listened well enough to spit back their same words, but then we would never know if real communication had taken place—i.e., "message sent, same message received." What you want to tell them is your understanding of what they said, not the same words. This is important because one word to you might mean something completely different to them. Really hearing means understanding the meaning of the message. In order to make certain I really heard my partner, I need to paraphrase back to them what my understanding of their message is and must use different words to accomplish that.

Continuing this example, the receiver might say, "What I'm hearing you say is that you're angry at me because you felt like you could count on me to be there at 5 p.m. to pick you up. And you're angry because I wasn't there when I said I would be there."

Next, check and see if the sender feels understood. And remember, understanding does not mean agreement. Understanding just means understanding. At this point, there's just one question that needs to be answered: Did the receiver correctly understand what the sender was saying? The receiver does not have to agree with the sender's point in any way. But did he understand the point the sender was trying to make?

If the sender does not feel understood, try again using different words. What hopefully happens is that when the receiver shares their understanding, the sender sees what the receiver missed or what they didn't communicate.

Here's a tip that will help you in this process: The sender is always the only one responsible for whether or not their partner understood them. One of the biggest mistakes people make in communicating with each other happens when the sender becomes aggravated because their partner isn't getting it. Then we put them down for not listening. Or we just keep saying the exact same thing over and over again—usually louder and louder. This kind of behavior is counter-productive. If they aren't getting it with the words you're using, do you really think they'll get it if you just say it louder and louder? Change your approach. If what you're doing isn't working, do something different.

Think about it. If I go to France and I don't speak French, but I ask a local for directions to a hotel in English, it wouldn't make any sense for me to get angry with them because they didn't understand me. And it would be ludicrous for me to say the same words over and over, and louder and louder, hoping each time that if I just say it loud enough, they'll understand me. That would be foolish. They'd most likely be insulted by my rude behavior and turn and walk away. I'd be frustrated, and on top of that I still wouldn't know how to get to the hotel. No one's happy, and I didn't get what I wanted or needed. It's often the same kind of scenario in relationships. Even though we may each be speaking English, we're still speaking a foreign language to some degree because we each have our own version of the same language.

If I'm the sender and I take full responsibility for being understood, I can't put any blame on the receiver for not understanding. It's up to me to communicate in such a way that they understand me. This is pure and simple diplomatic protocol—public relations with your most significant relation.

So the sender continues to send this one piece of information until they're certain the receiver understands them. The back-and-forth defining and refining of the problem contributes to its understanding.

Once the sender feels completely understood, they switch roles. The receiver becomes the sender and makes a statement to the new receiver (formerly the sender) that begins: "What I'm angry about is . . ." Then they go through the same steps described above. Once the new sender feels completely understood, they switch roles again and go on to the next emotion in this process.

From here on out, the process is exactly the same. The only thing that changes is the emotion they are talking about.

Here is the list of emotions the couple will talk about:

- "What I'm angry about is . . ."
- "What hurts the most is . . ."
- "What I regret most is . . ."
- "What I want is . . ."
- "You can count on me to . . ."

Sometimes people have difficulty with the "What I Regret Most" part. Let me give you some help in understanding the intention behind this part of the exercise so you can be more successful with it.

This particular message must be about the sender's own behavior. Not "I regret that you didn't pick me up." That is a message about their partner's behavior. An example of their own regret might be, "I regret that I asked you to pick me up. I probably should have asked a friend or just taken a cab. That way, I could have been more certain of having made my appointment on time."

After both partners have fully understood each other's feelings of regret, they next move into asking for what they want. Remember, keep your messages clear and concise.

"What I want is . . ." This is where you send a very clear message about specific, concrete things you want. It can't be nebulous. It can't be: "What I want is for you to love me." That is too nonspecific. "I want you to show your love for me by cooking dinner tonight"—now that's specific! Say anything you want. It doesn't mean you're going to get it from your partner. That's not the goal. The goal is communication. Whether or not your partner gives you what you want is totally up to them. Love is a gift, not a demand.

After both partners clearly understand each other's wants, it's time to move on to the last section.

"You can count on me to . . ." This is where you fill in the blank with what you can do to make sure your own needs are met. For example, "You can count on me (if I've been let down by you) to work at having more realistic expectations about your abilities to stay on task and then make decisions for myself so as not to set you up to disappoint me like this again." That's something you really can do to take better care of yourself and then enjoy the relationship more.

Or, the other person might say: "You can count on me to work at being more responsible for my commitments. I may not make it right away, but you can count on me to work on this."

Often, people are able to resolve their conflicts by just going through this process, even though it's not really a conflict-resolution tool. It's just a tool for learning how to communicate more effectively and more intimately. Most of the time, after the couple completes the "What I Want" section, they both realize they want the same thing. But they didn't know it because they weren't really listening to and understanding each other.

When you first start to do this process, it may feel awkward and goofy. That's normal because you're not used to it. No one in real life talks this way all of the time. People often tell me this is hard, but it just seems that way because it's new. Brushing your teeth is easy because you've done it almost all of your life. Are you right-handed? Try brushing your teeth with your left hand. Brushing with your left hand only seems hard because it's new. The more you practice, the easier it becomes. Should you talk this way to each other all the time? Heck no—people would think you were strange. This is only an exercise to help you both learn how to listen more accurately and more lovingly, and make certain in the process that each of you is addressing your significance needs.

Guidelines for Good Communication

1. When your partner is speaking to you, ask yourself: "Am I really listening to her right now?" Remind yourself that what your partner is saying right now is really important and that you really need to attend to what she is saying.

2. Remember to breathe.

3. Slow the conversation down. If you're talking too fast, you need to slow down what you're saying. If the conversation is going too fast for you to keep up, for whatever reason, identify that and work at slowing it down so you can both be heard and understood.

4. Make your point, clearly and concisely, then be quiet and listen. Ask your partner to paraphrase back to you what you just said to make certain that you have communicated clearly. Then invite your partner to share their views with you. Or vice versa.

5. If you're taking medication for your ADD, you need to be on your medication at that moment. Don't try to have a decent conversation unless you're on your medication. For the non-ADD person: Realize when the conversation is nonproductive because your partner is not on their medication. If they are not on their ADD medication, chances are the conversation won't go too well. If now is not a good time to work this out, postpone the conversation to a time when the ADD partner can be on their medication, like the next day or after they've had their medication in them for at least a half hour.

6. If the conversation begins to get antagonistic, take a break. Give yourselves permission to take a breather and then come back at a time when cooler heads will prevail.

7. Remember what's important in all good communication: *I want to get my idea across. I want to be heard.* What is the most loving and respectful way you can do that? And what can you do to make it more inviting for your partner to want to share with you?

8. Love is a choice, not a demand. Remember that your partner is only obligated to you as long as he or she wants to be. Avoid ultimatums.

9. When all else fails—or before it even gets close to that point—get the help of a professional who can impartially direct you through the process and teach both of you how to communicate better.

10. If you really love this person, be willing to do whatever it takes—in healthy ways—to make the relationship work. Evaluation. Medication. Therapy. Less work at the office. Doing the things you liked to do together when you first started dating . . . anything. It all helps. It all counts.

Follow these guidelines. Remember that effective communication can make or break a relationship. Both ADD and non-ADD couples can benefit from better, more open communication.

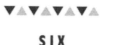

SIX

The Erratic Erotic Attention Span: Sexual Intimacy and ADD

Sexual intimacy can be one of the most wonderful aspects of a romantic relationship. When the relationship is going well, sex is a beautiful and pleasurable way for both partners to express their love for one another.

We talk a lot about sex in this country. Advertising campaigns designed around sex sell everything from cars to toothpaste. We talk about sex on the radio, on TV, in movies, and on the Internet. Sex is everywhere. You'd think we have very few hang-ups about sex since we talk about it so much. But when we do talk about sex, the content is more often bravado than factual. Our culture has many shameful feelings about sexuality and uses bravado as a way to hide that shame. Shame inhibits our ability to talk about sex factually, and in turn propagates both our ignorance and more shame. This is a vicious cycle.

Sexual intimacy is one of the most powerful human experiences. It can incorporate all realms of our being—physical, mental, emotional, and spiritual—at one cosmic moment.

We need to realize that we have a natural appetite for sex, just like we have an appetite for food or drink. Those appetites aren't good or bad. It's simply the way God made us. When it comes to our sexual appetite, it really isn't that much different from our appetite for food and drink, except that we *can* live without sex.

In a romantic relationship in which both partners have average sexual appetites, it makes no sense for them to "starve" themselves sexually. A major caveat to this, of course, would be if the couple is exercising sexual abstinence because of spiritual beliefs. Otherwise, *Eros*, or "erotic love," is one of the most beautiful mysteries of life that the two of you can share together. It's a remarkable way for each of you to express your love for one another. Plus, it's a powerful way to experience "into-me-see" (intimacy) in ways that words cannot even come close to expressing.

In fact, sex seems to be a very healthy part of normal metabolic processes in the brain. Sexual intimacy releases endorphins in the brain, which creates an experience of euphoria. Euphoria is the result of the metabolic change created by the release of endorphins. When both partners can experience this sexual euphoria together, they feel closer, more connected, and more loving toward each other. It's important for the longevity of their relationship for both partners to continue to experience the powerful bonding that takes place through sexual intimacy.

Of course, regardless of whether or not you have ADD, people can develop problems in their romantic relationship when there is a difference in sexual appetites.

When it comes to food appetites, some people like steak while others prefer lobster. Some people go for a plain ol' American hamburger. Any vegetarians in the crowd? Some people eat a little and some people eat a lot, it just depends upon your appetite. It's the same with sex. Everybody has their own appetite. That isn't a bad thing, but it does mean there are differences. Those differences can lead to problems if the couple doesn't spend time talking with each other about their needs and desires. They need to make certain the sexual needs of each are being met. If both partners aren't getting their sexual needs met, problems develop that can lead to hurt feelings, and possibly even affairs. Even though we talk about sex just about every place else—radio, TV, movies, books, and magazines—if it isn't being talked about in the bedroom, there will likely be problems.

If your husband isn't doing something sexually that you would like him to do, you've got to tell him what you would like and ask for it. If you don't talk about it, is he supposed to read you mind? Tell him, "I like it when you touch me this way," and then show him exactly what you mean. If you need to, take his hand in yours and demonstrate what it is that you like. If you like him nibbling on your ear, tell him and then demonstrate on his ear so he knows exactly what you're talking about. The only way he can really know what you want is for you to tell and show him.

Men, the same holds true for you. Your partner can't read your mind. You've got to let her know what you like too.

Being able to talk intimately about sex can be difficult if you haven't already mastered the art of talking and listening to each other about other subjects.

Obviously, if something doesn't feel good, you've got to talk about that too. If there is something that you want sexually that your partner doesn't want, you've got to discuss it. As I've mentioned before, love—especially erotic love—is a gift. Demanding that your partner give you a gift is not love. That's slavery.

Love invites sharing. Love respects boundaries. Love is gentle. Love is giving and receiving, not demanding and stealing.

The Effects of ADD on Sex

For a really good sexual relationship, each partner must take responsibility for their own sexual feelings, be able to communicate those feelings to their partner, and be able to clearly understand both their own and their partner's needs and feelings. But when ADD is part of the picture, it can cause difficulties in the bedroom just as it causes difficulties in other aspects of the relationship. In this first section we're going to look at how ADD may directly affect sexual intimacy. Then we'll look at some secondary effects it has. Later in this chapter, we'll look at how ADD medications affect sexual intimacy.

Throughout the general population, the two most common areas of sexual performance problems are the inability to come to orgasm and coming to orgasm too quickly. These are also the two most common problems in sexual performance when Attention Deficit Disorder is involved. There certainly can be many other factors creating problems in sexual intimacy other than just ADD. But if we're going to look at ADD in romance, we need to address the specific areas of sexuality affected by ADD.

1) Sex and Inattention

In a very basic sense, sex requires concentration. If you have difficulty staying on task in school or at work because of ADD, you might also have difficulty staying on task where sex is concerned.

We all too often think of our sexual organs as simply our genitalia. Technically speaking, our largest sex organ is probably our skin. You know . . . sensual touch. But the brain is the most important sex organ we've got because it's the brain that interprets and processes all of the messages from all other parts of the body, including "other" sex organs. Even though we know it feels good when we are touched somewhere on or near our genitalia, the actual sensation is experienced in our brain.

Naturally, when your mind is focused on sex, you become sexually aroused. That's just the way we were designed. But if your mind is wandering because ADD makes it difficult or impossible to stay focused, there could be some problems performing sexually.

Imagine yourself and your partner in a romantic embrace, when the moment is right and your sexual feelings begin to surge through your body. Just as things are starting to get good and the heat of passion is enveloping your body, you relax your mind and let it float off to wherever it takes you. That's all part of good sex. Unfortunately, your relaxed ADD mind may float off to all kinds of stuff, like the stack of bills on your desk that need to be paid, the dust on the dresser, or your daughter's cry from her bedroom down the hall. Just when things were going so well, your mind drifts too far off task, you lose focus, the feelings subside and . . . there are problems.

I remember talking with a young man at a conference I was teaching at. He shared with me the guilt and shame he experienced because of how ADD affects sexual intimacy between he and his wife. He described something similar to the previous scenario, though it hadn't affected his performance. He was still young and virile. He told me his wife had no idea of what was happening inside of him while they were making love, and he was afraid to tell her for fear of hurting her feelings.

When sexually intimate with his wife, in the midst of all their sexual bliss, his mind would drift off . . . to thinking about mowing the lawn or changing the oil in their car. His mind drifted off to just about anything but the love he was making to his wife at that moment. He felt so guilty that he wasn't able to focus on his bride—even in the passion of the moment. He felt as if he couldn't tell her for fear of hurting her feelings. That part of our brain which gives us the ability to think and create and love was also the very part of his brain that was sabotaging the joy and ecstasy of sexual communion with his wife.

So first there's the personal frustration of not being able to stay on task sexually. Then there's the embarrassment and shame he experiences from not being able to love his wife the way he would like to love her—in a fully attentive way. There's also the painful isolation he feels because he can't share his feelings with the most important person in his life for fear of hurting her. Besides the actual problem he is experiencing because of his ADD, there are now secondary problems—the frustration, shame, and isolation—which can compound and make things even worse if not addressed.

On more than one occasion, a woman has commented that she doesn't enjoy sex that much anymore because she senses her mate really isn't "present" with her even during sex. One woman told me she felt like a prostitute. Lacking any sense of her husband being present with her, she felt she was "just a piece of meat" to him. That's why the young man we were talking about a moment ago would never tell his wife what was going on. He would never want her to have to experience pain like that, although she might already be aware that something is wrong.

In terms of the mechanical aspects of sexual performance, it's fortunate for this young man that he has youth on his side. He is able to perform sexually without any effect on erection or orgasm. For older men, that might be a different story. As men age (although they continue to produce semen throughout their life) the length of time between ejaculations increases, and arousal and performance may require a greater ability to focus if he is to maintain erection and eventually ejaculate. As men get older, the ability to stay focused on arousal is of paramount importance. If a male can't stay focused, he may eventually become impotent. First because of the inability to stay on task during arousal, and secondly, because of psychological problems that men suffer because of decreased libido. Then, when performance anxiety sets in, that makes it even more difficult for him to perform. After enough experiences like that, "why even bother?" As you can see, this can be very debilitating

When ADD is present in males, difficulty staying on task can have a tremendously painful effect on the enjoyment of sexual intimacy for both partners, and can really affect a man's ability to perform sexually. Likewise, ADD in women presents sexual challenges as well. If a woman's ADD mind wanders off, she might not be able to naturally self-lubricate. It is possible that her ability to self-lubricate may be tied into her own sexual ego (just as a man's ability to maintain an erection may be tied to his sexual ego). Without lubrication, intercourse is likely to become painful—definitely decreasing one's desire for sexual intimacy. Fortunately, there are artificial lubrications available to compensate for this. There are certainly many other biological factors totally separate from ADD which may affect a woman's ability to naturally self-lubricate, but loss of focus on her own sexual feelings because her ADD mind drifts away can be major.

The most common problem of all for women with ADD who lose their focus during sex is inability to attain orgasm. Orgasmic response to stimuli is difficult when one's brain is not processing that stimuli completely. Literally, "the spirit is willing but the flesh is weak." This has nothing to do with the woman's desire for sex, her partner, or their intimate time together. It has to do with her ADD.

Research indicates that there is very little difference in the way that males and females experience sexual stimuli in their brains. Is it any wonder then that ADD affects both women and men in very similar ways in terms of sexual intimacy? Both women and men can have problems with arousal, and both can have problems with orgasmic response. Although the symptoms may be a bit different, the main problem is still the same: ADD and the inability to stay focused.

2) Sex and Hyperfocus

Sometimes ADD can cause a person to *hyperfocus*. If you will recall, hyperfocusing happens when the individual hyperfocuses on something because it is stimulating for them to do so. For a woman, hyperfocusing on the sexual and sensual feelings she has in her body during foreplay and sex will make sex much more enjoyable.

Women already are capable of multiple orgasms. Hyperfocusing on her sexual feelings can increase a woman's enjoyment of sex and increase orgasmic functioning. This is an instance in which ADD is actually beneficial.

But if a man has the hyperfocusing traits of ADD and becomes hyperfocused on the sexual and sensual feelings in his own body during foreplay and intercourse, he might be prone to early ejaculation—coming to orgasm and ejaculating when the process of sexual intimacy has barely begun. For a man, early ejaculation (previously know as premature ejaculation) can often lead to feelings of shame, guilt, and inadequacy because he is unable to satisfy his mate. And those negative feelings, of course, are not conducive to great sex. The downward emotional spiral that results from multiple experiences of early ejaculation can be completely demoralizing for a man.

Early ejaculation can be a sexual frustration for his mate as well. There she is, enjoying the moment, taking her time to enjoy every last ounce of sexual sensation she feels in her body. All of a sudden, before her sexual appetite has been satiated through orgasm, it's over. Often the woman will be understanding and nurturing towards her partner, which is nice and probably necessary for a man's frail sexual ego. But what about her needs? Talk about sexual frustration. It's one thing to go without satisfying one's sexual appetite. It's another thing entirely to step up to a glorious banquet table only to have someone clear the table just when you are about to sit down and eat.

Fortunately, there are things that can be done to compensate for the effects ADD has on sex.

First and foremost, there are medications (neurostimulants) to help people who daydream during sex stay on task. Maintaining focus will, in turn, help performance, as you are better able to consistently experience the sexual feelings in your body and stay with those feelings until blissful climax. Like any other part of your life—work, school, or play—you need your brain working for you when making love as well. After all, your brain *is* the most important sexual organ in your body.

Good communication is paramount in having good sex. As we saw in Chapter Five, learning how to talk with each other in nonthreatening ways increases the quality of the relationship. Applying good communication skills when we talk about sex can only make sex better (unless of course you are *talking* about sex more than you are *having* sex). Again, medication can often help people who have ADD communicate better.

If there are problems with early ejaculation, there are medications like Prozac, Zoloft, and Luvox that may be helpful in retarding ejaculation so that sexual intimacy can be prolonged before the male ejaculates. Using desensitization creams, which your doctor can recommend, or using double condoms may help in decreasing the sensitivity of the penis. Talking with your partner about your feelings instead of harboring guilt and shame may also help by decreasing performance anxiety. There are also many other ways to sexually satisfy your mate other than just coming on cue. Caress her, fondle her, massage her. Let your mind run wild. Ask her what she likes and do that for her. Don't throw in the towel just because you're done. I remember while growing up, my parents taught us to stay at the dinner table until the last person is finished. That's just good manners. It's the same for sex.

There are so many other things you can do to help make your sex life better, such as having a thorough medical checkup to make certain there isn't some other medical issue causing problems. Counseling, sex therapy, maybe just time away from your kids so you can finally have some peace and quiet together—these can all help to make sexual intimacy more fulfilling and satisfying.

3) Sex, Impatience, and Impulsivity

People who have ADD can often be impatient, and their impatience can negatively affect the splendors of foreplay. Their concept of foreplay may consist of: "Hey baby, let's do it!" That's not very romantic.

Once again, the importance of medication for treatment of ADD cannot be overemphasized. When your prefrontal cortex is properly medicated, you have a much better chance of not feeling so restless. You can be more patient. You can slow the process down and enjoy the ride instead of arriving at your final destination faster than a speeding bullet. There is lots to see and feel and do along the way. And sometimes the process of getting there can actually be more fun than your final destination. So if you're restless and impatient, you may find that your ADD medication can have a wonderful effect on your sex life. ADD medications can help curb your restlessness and decrease your impatience, which can make for much better sex.

Although impatience can cause problems in romantic relationships, there is a greater potential for problems when the ADD characteristic of impulsivity is involved. Impulsivity can sometimes lead to affairs.

Most of us, whether or not we are involved in a monogamous relationship, see people whom we find attractive. And that's very normal. But when one person in the relationship has ADD and the poor impulse control that sometimes comes along with it, that person may be more likely to act on those feelings of sexual attraction. As you can imagine, that impulsive act can destroy their relationship with the one they love.

Time and time again, we hear stories of people who have impulsively had a sexual affair and regretted it with every ounce of their being—the destruction it causes, the pain that results, and the chaos that ensues. If you know you have a problem with impulsiveness and you want to keep your romance alive with the love of your life, take every step necessary to keep that relationship untainted. Take your medication, see a therapist, go to twelve-step groups devised to help people with this kind of impulsivity, and pray like there's no tomorrow to guard against your impulsiveness.

There are many different shadings to ADD symptoms, and many other life values that come into play as someone with ADD interacts with life. Just because your partner has hyperactive/impulsive ADD doesn't mean they're going to have an affair. Just because you have hyperactive/impulsive ADD doesn't mean you're going to have an affair or even be tempted to have an affair. There are so many other factors to life—and to you. But it's necessary to examine how ADD *may* affect romance. I'd hate to see you miss out on a fabulous life of love and romance because you came to believe that everyone who has ADD will have affairs. That's just not true. There is so much more to a person than just their ADD.

4) ADD, Sex, and Unresolved Conflicts

Generally speaking, when someone is angry with someone else, they don't want to have sex with that person. Anger takes away from the passion of the moment. Unfortunately, in relationships involving an ADD partner, there can be lots of unresolved conflicts—chronic, low-grade anger hiding under the surface—that really decrease the chances of creating sexual intimacy.

Any of the topics we've discussed so far in this book can result in long-standing anger about unresolved issues. For example, if your partner said he would pick you up at 5 p.m. and left you stranded at work instead, you're probably not going to be in the most romantic mood when you get home that night. If you're angry and frustrated because your partner never lets you get a word in edgewise, or has suddenly stopped writing you love notes or letting you know she cares, you're probably not going to feel like making love. If your husband was just fired from his fifth job because he couldn't control himself and impulsively "told off" yet another supervisor, you're probably going to feel both angry and worried—again, not the greatest prescription for romance.

Unfortunately, any of the many negative effects ADD can have on a relationship may result in the partners feeling emotionally distant, then sexually distant. Maybe they're scared of what will happen in terms of financial security. Fear certainly can decrease one's libido in a hurry. All the more reason to make certain that ADD doesn't get in the way of you both having a great relationship—a relationship that is alive with romance, passion, and really great sex.

5) ADD and the Need for Novel Sex

"Variety is the spice of life." We've all heard that phrase. And variety—change in positions, places, and settings—can contribute to a better sex life. But for the purposes of this book, variety and novelty are two different things. ADD and the need for novel sex is not all that common. But there are some people who struggle with this. Again, this is not a common problem in ADD, but it does sometimes happen.

Some couples may run into difficulty when one partner has what some geneticists are calling the "novelty gene." There may be an actual genetic "anomaly" for some people in which a certain dopamine receptor in their brain causes them to constantly desire, or actually need, newer, more novel types or higher levels of stimulation. Whatever it is they're doing, they have a constant need for novelty. Sexually, they may search out "novel" ways to have sex. When the novelty wears off, then they need to "kick it up a notch" in order for that activity to provide stimulation. They need a sense of novelty in order to be able to perform sexually.

For example, let's say the first time Robin (who seeks novelty) and Victor had sexual intercourse, they used the missionary position, and sex in that position was fabulous for both of them. After a while, it didn't seem to be as fabulous for Robin because it lost its novelty. So they experimented and found something they both liked that was new and stimulating. After the novelty of that new sexual experience wore off, Robin needed to move up to the next level of novelty for sex to be satisfying. After a while, as their novel experiences got moved up too many notches for Victor, "novelty" became something way outside his comfort zone. Victor began to avoid Robin's sexual advances towards him for fear of what she might be suggesting next.

When one partner needs novelty for sexual intimacy to be stimulating, that can be very frustrating for both partners. The partner with the "novelty gene" may have a difficult time getting their partner to continually move up to higher levels of novelty. And without that novelty, they are not able to satisfy their own sexual appetite. The other partner might find themself being asked to do sexual things they are not comfortable doing—things that may actually scare them or run counter to their religious or moral values. At that point, the disparity between their sexual appetites can become so immense that the couple ceases to be sexually intimate and both partners become sexually frustrated.

ADD and the need for novel sex is something that most likely will need to be dealt with in couples counseling and with the aid of a good psychiatrist. You'll definitely need a professional who understands the complexities of this problem and who can provide an emotionally safe and nurturing therapeutic environment to work through these problems. The last thing you need at this point is someone judging you and shaming you. That won't help anything. In fact, it may only drive you to having to deal with it on your own, alone and without good guidance and direction.

The Effects of ADD Medication on Sex

Most likely, if you've got ADD and are receiving medical treatment, you're taking a neurostimulant. The most commonly prescribed neurostimulants are Ritalin, Dexedrine, and Adderall. People often find that by taking their medication regularly (as prescribed), their sex life improves. That's because their untreated

ADD was probably negatively affecting their sex life in at least some of the ways we've discussed in this chapter. Theoretically, when you take medicine to fix the neurobiological problems in your brain, you should also be fixing the problems your untreated brain was causing.

Usually, that's what happens. Often after a person begins medical treatment for their ADD, they feel like a new person. Sex becomes better because they're finally able to be present with their partner and focus on their partner's sexual needs, as well as their own sexuality, much more clearly. They're better able to bond and connect emotionally during and after making love. They're on a more stable course emotionally, which makes for better romance and sex with their partner. And they're usually handling their life better in general, which makes them feel more peaceful and more giving in their relationship.

Generally, most people are not going to have any negative side effects from their ADD medication, but some people do experience side effects. In that case, it's very important to talk to your doctor about those side effects immediately. Whether or not you should stop taking your medication because of a negative side effect ought to first be discussed with your physician. Your physician may want to stop the medication immediately, or they may want to taper you off slowly. That decision will be based on the physician's knowledge of you and the medication you are taking.

Sometimes, people will have some unpleasant side effects while their body is adjusting to the medication. I know when I first started taking Ritalin for my ADD, I had headaches for a while. I talked with my physician, and he suggested I take something like Advil or Tylenol until my body adjusted. He was right. The headaches only lasted a couple weeks and then they were over. No big deal, but there was an adjustment phase my body was going through.

Different medications have different side effect profiles. Your physician should know which side effects are common and which ones are not. If you're experiencing problems, you've got to talk with your physician about them because it may be just a transition phase you're going through. Ultimately, medication is supposed to make your life better, not worse. If for some reason you don't respond to the prescription you were given, there are several other medication approaches that can be utilized to treat your ADD. So if one medication doesn't work, have hope. There are others your doctor can work with.

Occasionally, people will have a bad reaction to a neurostimulant. Those reactions can include temporary impotence. But that kind of reaction is rare and it is only temporary. Once off the medication, the impotency goes away. If you should happen to develop impotency, see a doctor and ask him or her to switch you to a different ADD medication. It's unlikely that you would have the same kind of reaction on one of the other ADD medications.

On the other hand, if a male is prone to early ejaculation because of untreated ADD, that problem can become even worse when his ADD is medicated and he is able to focus even more on his sexual feelings. If that should happen, his doctor might want him to try a different neurostimulant. Or his doctor might want to add to his neurostimulant a low dose of another kind of medication called a Serotonin Selective Reuptake Inhibitor (SSRI) such as Prozac, Zoloft, and Luvox. That combination—neurostimulant and SSRI—could help him stay on task but also help to decrease the sensitivity of his penis so he's less likely to have early ejaculation.

Women usually don't experience any negative side effects from neurostimulants that affect their sexuality. They may have some headaches while adjusting to the medication, but that's usually transitory. A wonderful benefit of the increased focus gained by taking medication is an increased ability to not only achieve orgasm, but oftentimes an increase in the ability to experience multiple orgasms. So far, there aren't too many women who consider that to be a *negative* side effect.

In some cases, doctors start their ADD patients on a course of medication other than neurostimulants. They might start them on SSRIs, which, as we've noted before, are a special class of anti-depressants. Remember, the medications that physicians use to treat one problem can often be used to treat others as well. So even if you're not depressed, your physician may want to use that medication to treat another part of your brain.

Some SSRIs are known to involve some frustrating side effects, including decreased libido and decreased sexual performance. This may affect a man's ability to obtain and maintain an erection. Besides the decreased desire for sex, it may also cause a decrease in a woman's ability to lubricate. If this occurs, talk with your physician about these kinds of side effects. Remember, medication is supposed to make your life better, not worse. Maybe you need a different medication. Maybe you just need an adjustment in the dose you are taking. Maybe you need an additional prescription to better balance your brain. Talk with your doctor.

The side effects we just talked about may actually be benefits in some ways for other people.

Let's say a couple is prone to conflicts and arguments, but they really love each other and are working at their relationship. Still, one person seems more susceptible to the pain their conflicts create. A physician may want to prescribe an SSRI so that partner can become more emotionally "thick-skinned"—one of the side effects which often accompanies SSRIs. The SSRI may help to dull their emotions (so they're not as emotionally present in the relationship) *a little* so they can better cope with the stress of ongoing conflicts, recover from them faster, and be in a better frame of mind. A possible negative side effect of SSRIs—the dulling of emotions—may actually become the effect needed to make things better in a relationship.

There are all kinds of medications that can be used for different aspects of ADD. Plus, there are other over-the-counter medications that might also help. Natural supplements like Ginkgo Biloba and

St. John's Wort have been recognized by many physicians to be beneficial in helping to treat sexual problems associated with ADD. Both Ginkgo Biloba and St. John's Wort extracts come from plants of the same names and are available without a prescription at most drugstores. What should you use? Ask your physician.

Here are ten things to consider in making sexual intimacy better for you and your partner.

1. If you're ADD, take your medication. Usually that will make things better before, during, and after sex.

2. Learn how to communicate effectively both outside and inside the bedroom. Learn how to share your feelings, your wants, and desires (in supportive and loving ways) through direct communication with your mate. You can't expect them to read your mind. You've got to tell them.

3. Recognize boundaries. This is a very important part of good sex. Sexual intercourse is one of the most intimate experiences, if not the most intimate experience, available to us as humans. It requires a lot of trust and faith in your partner to let them so deeply into your heart. When we're sexually intimate, we're also emotionally vulnerable. If your partner sets a boundary, respect that boundary. Set boundaries for yourself that you need in order to feel safe and comfortable. Then, within the safety of the structure you have created, relax and enjoy one another.

4. Relax. Sex is supposed to be fun, not work. Experiment with each other. Touch here. Taste there. Play with each other. Become lost in the moment and enjoy the thrill and the ecstasy of sensuality.

5. Try to avoid getting into a rut. Sometimes we get into the same old routine of working all day, dinner and dishes at

night, and then, if you both have strength after working all day, you jump in the sack, turn out the lights, and catch a quickie before you go to sleep. It becomes commonplace. Every time, the same old thing. If sex is less exciting than it used to be, try different positions. Make love someplace new in the house, or somewhere outside. Of course, you'll want to use caution so as not to offend or embarrass someone else. But there are plenty of open spaces out there. You never know what a little change in scenery can do for your sex life. There's nothing wrong with developing a pattern, but just add a little zing once in a while.

6. Making love is more than sex. Sex is relatively simple: put tab "A" into slot "B" and *voilá*, you're done. Making love is so much more than this. Making love begins when you get up in the morning. It happens throughout your day and deep into the night. Making love is how you respect each other, care for each other, and stand up for each other. It's believing in each other and supporting each other's dreams. The true beauty of sexual intimacy should be the culmination of making love throughout the day.

7. Foreplay is a good thing. In the media hype that sex gets, the focus tends to be on the act of sexual intercourse. At most, there's the briefest depiction of making out beforehand, or cuddling afterwards. There's so much more to experience, so much more to foreplay. Unfortunately, most people don't even have a clue about really good foreplay.

   In my college sex therapy classes we were required to keep a sex journal as part of our homework. We were to experiment with our mates and try different touches on different parts of our bodies and then write about our experiences. I was amazed to find when I focused on my entire body and the sensations I felt during foreplay that there is so much more to sexual feelings than one's genitals. I've met people who can have orgasmic experiences without having a "traditional orgasm," all by focusing on other parts of the body that respond to sensual touch. Try it. You'll like it.

8. Schedule *spontaneity* into your sex life. At first that sounds like a total contradiction, but think about it. These days in two-income households where both partners are rushing here and there trying to get everything done that they are supposed to, sometimes sexual intimacy takes a back seat. One of you or even both of you need to schedule some time to spontaneously surprise your lover with a sexual treat. Schedule spontaneity? Maybe it's come down to that. So what? Make it happen. Even if it's just a "nooner" or a quickie, make time for romance and sexual intimacy. Even if you have to schedule it.

9. Seek professional help. If there are problems for the two of you, sexually, and the things I've listed above don't seem to help, seek the help and advice of a professional. See your physician. See a therapist trained in sex therapy who also knows a lot about ADD. Do whatever it takes for both of you to have wonderful, satisfying, playful sex. This is too important a part of romance to avoid or forget about. There are many steps you can take to make things better. Push past the embarrassment and shame and go get the help you need.

10. Last but not least: If you're not in a monogamous relationship, by all means, practice safe sex.

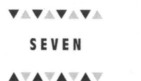

SEVEN

The Positive Attributes of ADD in a Romantic Relationship

While I was writing this book, I had to make a brief trip from my home in California to teach about ADD in adults at an international conference in Washington, D.C. Usually I fly both ways, but on this particular trip I decided to go there by train and then fly home at the end of the conference. It would make my trip much longer, but I love riding on trains, and I knew the ride would give me some much-needed quiet time to get some work done—some place away from phones, traffic, and the appointments I rush to on a daily basis. The only drawback was how much I would miss my wife, Terri, who also has ADD. Although she encouraged me to take the opportunity to get away and get some rest and relaxation—and some important work done—she also knew how much we would miss each other.

That first night in the sleeper car on the train, when I was tired and all alone, I opened my suitcase and found a stack of greeting cards from my wife and my daughters. There was one marked for me to open every day of the week I would be gone. They had also enclosed photographs which I promptly taped to the wall with a

Band-Aid borrowed from the cabin steward. As I read and re-read the cards throughout the week, it was obvious that my wife had hand-picked each card especially for me. The messages in the cards fit either me or her perfectly. Terri had put a lot of time and effort into making me feel loved on that trip. It was a wonderful experience. Terri and I both try to do something like this for each other when we have to be away for any extended length of time.

So far in this book, we've been focusing on the difficulties ADD creates in an intimate relationship—and there are many. But people with ADD also have many positive traits—because of their ADD—that make them wonderful partners, and that's what I'd like for us to look at now.

Of course, you don't have to have ADD to send cards or love notes to your partner. But people with ADD often hyperfocus on romance and are able to come up with some wonderfully creative ways of expressing their feelings of love. In this case, my wife had drawn upon some of the card-exchanging experiences we'd shared during our courtship—experiences that helped our love grow and develop even years after the initial infatuation settled down. She was utilizing a very ADD-influenced activity that she had seen and used during the courtship phase . . . and then, *by choice*, continued using it to strengthen the love we already have.

I remember when we were first dating I was hyperfocused on romance. I pulled out all the stops and did every romantic thing in the book—special dinners, candlelight, soft music, weekends at the coast, love notes on the windshield of her car, you name it. Luckily, by this time, I understood enough about my ADD and had it under control through medication so that I could enjoy the fabulous feelings of romance but still think clearly and not act too impulsively when it came to making important decisions.

During this courting phase, Terri went on a trip with some friends. This was a cruise that had been planned for quite a while, and she was very excited about it. I knew I was going to really miss her. And I definitely did not want her to forget about *me* during her trip. So I handed a stack of greeting cards to her roommate and asked her to dole them out to Terri, giving her one each day. Terri was totally surprised and delighted by my thoughtfulness, wrought out of my ADD hyperfocus on romance. And it was this act of kindness and love that she remembered and then implemented to make me feel loved and significant to her when I was away on my train trip to Washington.

And it worked. Every time I saw those cards, I fell more deeply in love and missed her even more. Even though neither of us are hyperfocused on romance these days—what with work, kids, church, and everything else—we still have a plethora of romantic experiences from which we can draw to nurture our romance and keep the love alive. It's so much more fun than barely sustaining our love life by getting trapped in the hectic schedules we both maintain. *We actively choose to use* the romance skills we learned previously in life to nurture our love today. We don't wait around hoping those feelings and actions will just naturally happen again. We take a pro-active approach to nurturing our relationship.

During the courtship phase of a romantic relationship, people with ADD are hyperfocused on romance and are continually showering their beloved with gifts and attention out of a frantic need to self-medicate with endorphins. But when ADD is diagnosed and appropriately medicated, those same behaviors that helped bring the two of you together can be used *by choice* to help the love grow in a relationship.

That phrase "by choice" is so important. Because mature love is a choice. A love that is strong enough to last a lifetime is a *choice*, not a *feeling*. Feelings can come and go, depending on many factors. But real love is a choice. Too often we think of love as only a feeling, but it is so much more. Love is also a verb, which implies action, an action you choose to take though a conscious decision. Love is more than those intense feelings we feel during the initial attraction between two people. Love is a commitment you make, and it's a commitment that requires action. Even in this relationship-challenged culture we live in today, most wedding vows promise "until death do us part"—not "until the intense feelings of love fade away." To the traditional wedding vows of "in sickness and in health, for richer or poorer," perhaps we should add "regardless of how I feel."

In any love story you've ever heard, there's always a hurdle for the lovers to overcome. In *Romeo and Juliet*, for example, it's the feud between the Capulets and the Montagues. It took action for Romeo and Juliet to push past everything so they could be together. If a love story touches your heart, it does so because one or both of the partners take some kind of action. They don't just sit there in love doing nothing. That kind of relationship would be of little interest to anyone—possibly even to themselves.

Remember, love is a verb. If you really love someone, you have to love them actively.

We tend to believe that feelings of love are supposed to come first, and that those feelings will then motivate us to take action. That's usually what happens in the courting process. We see someone across a crowded room, we are intensely attracted to that person, and we're suddenly ready to sweep them off their feet and whisk them away for a lifetime of romance. Feelings first, actions second.

After the honeymoon phase of a relationship is over, *real life* can be very different from that. Here's a radical thought. In real life, we need to act on our love first—especially when our love is devoid of feelings in the moment—if we want to experience those feelings and have them continue throughout the life of the relationship. With mature love, actions come first, then the feelings will follow. If I don't have the loving feelings that I want in a relationship, I need to take action—like the ADD person that I am—and *plan* something, *create* something, *make something happen*. I need to take action to remedy the situation. If I choose to just sit around and wait for that loving feeling to come back, it might never happen. But if I take action to demonstrate to my partner how much I love her, then chances are, those feelings of love will return.

I need to approach the relationship with actions first, feelings second. This is based in very sound psychological theory. If we invest in something (like the love relationship with our mate), we raise our commitment level to that thing. By taking action and investing time, energy, thoughts, and feelings, we are raising our level of commitment and doing the very things that can bring our love back to life. When we do this, what we are really doing is investing *ourselves* in the relationship. Of course, this concept will only work if you are *choosing* to invest yourself. It will not work if you feel you're being forced to invest yourself.

In many ways it's very much like investing money in the stock market. First you check out the different kinds of stocks. You make your investment and then you watch the paper each day to see how your investment is doing. You could play the stock market with play money forever as a way to dabble without getting burned, and that can be fun, but when you have invested actual currency into the stock, there's a sense of excitement. It's much the same with investing ourselves in our most significant adult relationship. The old phrase "it takes money to make money" is also true in lifelong love relationships. It takes love actions to make love feelings grow. It is an investment in you. It is an investment in your partner. And, it's an investment in the relationship itself.

Not too long ago, I was driving home from a business trip to Sacramento. It was late at night and I was exhausted. I was looking forward to getting home and unwinding from yet another hectic day of facilitating therapy, travel, and teaching. When I called Terri from the road to let her know I was on my way, she told me she had just come down with a cold and wasn't feeling well. We had no medicine in the house for flu or colds. I empathized with her for a while over the phone and told her I'd be home within an hour.

Tired as I was, I stopped at the next all-night market I saw to buy her some cold medicine. She hadn't asked me to do this, and I'm sure she could have waited until morning and picked something up on her way in to work. But I love my wife, and I knew this medicine would help her feel better. I also knew that this relatively small action would make her feel my love for her more than almost anything I could say. This was an action I made specifically for her.

While I was in the market I saw a little stuffed bunny on a shelf in the floral department. My wife collects bunnies. She absolutely loves them. So I bought it for her. It was not an extravagant purchase, but I knew she would enjoy it. I also got a bunch of red carnations (her favorite, next to tulips) while I was in the floral department. ADD spur-of-the-moment purchases. Done not out of ADD impulsiveness, but inspired by ADD hyperfocus on romance.

It was really kind of funny when I got to the checkout stand. The clerk asked me what terrible thing I had done to be in the doghouse—having to buy flowers and gifts at that time of night. The clerk was both shocked and amazed to learn that I had not done anything wrong, and that this old married man just wanted to express his love to his wife and let her know with both words and actions how much he cared for her.

I got home at one o'clock in the morning with a cute little bunny and flowers to cheer my wife up, plus some cold medicine she really needed, but hadn't asked for. Terri recognized these items for exactly what they were—signs of my deep and enduring love for her.

I hadn't relied on feelings. I relied on actions to show her my love and then received the benefit of warm, loving feelings as a result of my giving.

Maybe you remember back to a time during the courtship phase of your romance when you burst into your lover's office, interrupted her on the phone, and whisked her away for an afternoon in the park. Impulsive. Romantic. Well, you could now—by choice— plan for that exact same excursion and surprise your partner all over again. Only maybe this time, you can call the office manager in advance and notify her of your plans, and make sure your partner doesn't have any important meetings scheduled for that afternoon. That way you'll still be able to enjoy the thrill of being with your partner during the afternoon, but you'll be making a more responsible choice to spend that time with her instead of acting on impulse born from your personal need for endorphins.

When the honeymoon phase is over, you'll need to remember the actions you took when you were hyperfocused on romance. Borrow from that rich history of loving behaviors to find ways to minister to the heart of your lover today.

Creativity

People with ADD have been among the most creative people in the history of humankind. We know through their biographies that Edison, Bell, Einstein, Lincoln, and Churchill probably had ADD (though undiagnosed) and used their creativity—whether it was inventing technology or creating world policies—to change the course of history. People who have ADD often have an abundance of creativity—creativity that can be used in the active expression of romantic love.

Creativity can also come in handy when trying to solve problems. People with ADD can come up with incredible solutions for some complex problems. Solutions that their partner may never even dream of. Why? It's that creative ADD process that happens when several thoughts—all being entertained simultaneously—collide in the brain and something new develops. A brand-new thought, a unique solution to a particular problem.

I remember a TV commercial years ago in which one person was mindlessly walking down the street eating a chocolate candy bar while another person was mindlessly walking up the street eating peanut butter out of a jar. By chance, they bumped into each other, accidentally mixing their two favorite snacks together. In the process, a new taste treat was formed (a famous peanut butter and chocolate candy bar), something that neither had ever thought of before.

That's a great example of serendipity—of something happening by accident that works out quite well. It is also a great example of how the creative process happens in the mind of the person who has ADD.

When they turn their attention to their romantic partner, people with ADD can be extremely creative. But showing love doesn't always have to be on a grandiose scale. It's being creative in the little day-to-day things that can often really make a difference in a relationship. And sometimes you have to use your creative thinking to realize how best to show love to your partner.

Not too long ago, my wife left home early in the morning for work, with a long drive ahead of her. But when she was only a few blocks from our home, her car started to make a terrible noise. She turned around and came back. Terri asked me if I'd take a look at her car to see what was wrong, so I jacked it up and saw that one of her tires was in bad shape. When I went to put on her spare, it was flat. Naturally, I got in my car and drove her tire over to the gas station. By the time I came home and put on her spare, I realized I would be late for work. So I called in and left a message with my office. But before I did go to work, I checked every tire on my wife's car—just so she would know the other tires were fine and she could drive with confidence in the safety of her car that day. The real creativity in this example was not so much checking her tires as it was creatively rearranging my work schedule that day to accommodate choosing to show Terri my love for her in a concrete way that would mean a lot to her.

When we show our partners we love them, we need to show them in a way that makes *them* feel loved, which can be very different from what makes *us* feel loved.

For example, when I took all four tires off my wife's car so I could check them for safety, she really appreciated that. She hates dealing with cars. You might not immediately think that changing a tire is an act of love, but I knew my wife would feel my love through that action.

On the other hand, if she were to show her love for me by getting my car fixed, it wouldn't mean all that much to me because I don't mind working on cars. But when Terri gives me a loving, full-body massage at the end of a really hard day, that means the world to me.

Loyalty and Charisma

Many people who have ADD are extremely loyal. Even in the midst of turmoil in a relationship, they often have the tenacity to hang in there and not give up. ADD people can also be amazingly quick to forgive. Because of their sensitivity, they can be generous beyond measure, patient, understanding, and kind.

People with ADD are often very charismatic because of their vast life experiences derived from searching for the next stimulating encounter. They have an incredible knowledge base. They know interesting tidbits of information about a lot of different things. In addition, since learning (not necessarily school!) stimulates them, that knowledge base continues to grow throughout a lifetime. And being knowledgeable is a very attractive trait.

Empathy

People with ADD can be extremely warm-hearted and empathetic beyond belief. They can often zone in on their partner's feelings and know what their partner is feeling before their partner does. Because of their empathy and warm-heartedness, people with ADD can be very compassionate—giving the shirt off their back without a second thought, knowing the need and wanting to help.

Perhaps this empathy and compassion grow out of their own lifetime of pain. They have been so humbled in their own experiences, they are less likely to be judgmental. They know. They've been there. And so they reach out their hands and their hearts to comfort and encourage.

Intuition

Another fabulous gift many ADD people have developed and finetuned over a lifetime is intuition. They had to develop intuition as a way to cope with the challenges ADD creates for them because of their inattention. Since they may not have been attending at times that it was crucial for them to pay close attention, they learned how to size up situations, conversations, and people relatively quickly to avoid embarrassment or harm.

It's almost like people with ADD have had to develop a second sense to know how and what to do in many different situations. They've learned how to quickly figure out what other people are thinking or doing and what they need to do to take care of themselves. That's why they can often "sense" something accurately, long before anyone else does.

And that kind of insight can be very beneficial in a relationship. Often, they may be able to sense, through intuition, what the core issues are in a conflict and use that information to negotiate resolution more quickly.

Fun-Seeking

People with ADD can come up with some of the most creative ways to have fun. They like having a good time—"stimulation is my friend." And they can be an awful lot of fun to be with. They can open doors to new worlds, new views of life, new experiences for their partners through ADD-inspired creativity.

"Never a dull moment" can take on a whole new and wonderful meaning because of that desire to have fun. They don't do well with boredom in general, so they have a lifetime of experiences entertaining themselves and others when things get too boring. They're natural experts at it. And the fun side of ADD can be a tremendous boon to romantic relationships, because among other things, romance needs to be fun!

One of the first things I suggest to couples who come to see me with relationship or marital problems is that they just take some time off and spend it with each other. Stay away from the minefields associated with ongoing conflicts. Go play. Get to know each other again. Have fun. Get back in touch with all the wonderful things about each other that brought the two of you together in the first place. Remember how you showed your love to each other when you were first dating. It worked back then, and there's a good chance those same kinds of behaviors and thoughtfulness will also work now to rekindle your love for each other. Those kinds of *actions* may be exactly what it takes to bring back those *feelings* again.

I know one couple who kept those feelings alive in part by acting out their fantasies with each other. This was their own way of having fun. For example, Tim had always had a fantasy of picking up a girl in a bar and taking her home to have sex with her. Now, Tim was happily married to Julie and would *never* have picked up a woman in a bar. In addition, hanging out at bars and having one-night stands were completely outside his religious beliefs. He knew it and Julie knew it. Still, it was a fantasy that stayed with him, and he shared his fantasy with his wife.

One day, they went to a bar—separately. Julie arrived first, then Tim came into the bar a bit later. He spotted his wife across the room, introduced himself as if he had never met her before and asked to join her, and then bought her a drink.

After having a drink and telling each other a bit about themselves, he asked her back to his place. She agreed. So they went back to "his place" and had a wonderfully romantic and sexy evening together. The only reality check they faced in the morning—unlike what Tim would have faced if he had ever acted out this fantasy with a stranger—was that there was no embarrassment or hurt feelings for each other. There were no awkward excuses and exits to make. Plus, the one-night stand was turning out perfect—they were both very pleased with who they were waking up with. The only real drawback was that Julie's car was still at the bar and they had to go back and pick it up. A small price compared to the fun they had acting out Tim's fantasy.

It was a night Tim and Julie will never forget. And it was a night in which the *actions* they took certainly had a positive impact on their *feelings* for each other.

Just like Tim and Julie, when our relationships hit the doldrums, we have choices to make. We might not decide to act out a sexual fantasy, but we all have the freedom and the ability to take some action to improve our relationship. And one way to improve that relationship is to have some fun. ADD partners are wonderful mates when it comes to having fun.

Just as you enjoy people who are active and energetic and fun to be around, so does your partner. And given the gifts of ADD and its positive attributes, you have the ability to be even more active and energetic and exciting than most people. So use that gift. Use your ADD to its best advantage.

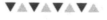

EIGHT

Making Your Love Last

Remember Annie and Bob Wilson, the unhappy couple we met in Chapter One? Annie and Bob both had ADD—and boy, did it cause problems in their relationship. These were two people who loved each other dearly, but their untreated ADD just tripped them up every time they turned around. They were argumentative, impulsive, and disorganized, and they absolutely seemed to crave conflict. Their lives and their relationship were just in shambles— and all because of their undiagnosed and untreated ADD and co-existing conditions.

Here's the flip side of the coin, so to speak.

I'd like you to meet Scott and Diane. Scott is a lab technician and Diane is a social worker. Both are in their early forties.

Like Annie and Bob, Scott and Diane both have ADD. They also have three children with ADD. But through diagnosis and treatment, they have not only worked through their ADD issues (and continue to work through those issues on a daily basis), they have also learned how to use the gifts that come with ADD to make their lives and their romantic relationship satisfying and fulfilling.

Scott and Diane have a loving, stable home life and a rock-solid relationship. Are they the "perfect" couple, the couple who is blissful every single second with never a raised voice or hurt feeling? No. That kind of relationship only exists in movies or novels. Every couple has squabbles at one time or another. That's reality. But Scott and Diane have learned how to make the best of their lives and how to continually nourish their romance and friendship. Their relationship is an example we could all learn from.

Scott and Diane were diagnosed as having ADD long after they became adults. In fact, their ADD wasn't diagnosed until after they were married. Neither of them had suffered seriously as a result of their ADD, but they did have some ADD-related problems and weren't working, or living, up to their potential.

Diane came from a family of fourteen children. Her biological father was an alcoholic and was out of her life before she was three years old. It was her stepfather who encouraged her to go to college. She had done fairly well academically through high school and decided to take his advice. While at college, Diane went to see a counselor for some help. She had always sensed that something wasn't quite right with her, but she couldn't put her finger on it. She had always been involved with extracurricular activities like the drama club, the yearbook, and the pep squad, and she always got good grades. Still, as far back as she could remember, school had always been extremely difficult for her. She had always had lots of friends, and yet, she felt "stupid" around them because she didn't understand things they were talking about. She told the counselor she didn't feel very smart, that she had difficulty concentrating and remembering things. "It's like something isn't connecting in my brain," she said. But the counselor told her nothing was wrong. Unconvinced, Diane next sought the help of a psychiatrist. Even he said, "You're fine. Don't worry about it." So, Diane let it go and went on with her education and earned her Master of Social Work degree and eventually licensing as a Licensed Clinical Social Worker (LCSW).

Unlike Diane, Scott, who came from a family of three children, did have trouble with academics. He had no overt behavioral problems, but he always had problems with his schoolwork. Like Diane, he was always busy in high school, involved in student government and other extracurricular activities. After high school, Scott went on to college, but it took him six years to earn a four-year Bachelor of Arts degree because he often felt overwhelmed by the academics. He took a semester off several times during his college career because of that draining sense of being overwhelmed.

Scott and Diane met when they were both working in a hospital. They belonged to the same employee after-work social group and enjoyed getting to know each other as friends. They both had a strong Christian faith and attended the same church. A few years after their friendship began, they became romantically involved.

During their courtship, both Scott and Diane became hyperfocused. In this particular case, because they knew they were hyperfocused on romance but were also trying to establish a strong foundation for their relationship, the hyperfocusing didn't cause any serious problems. In fact, it was enjoyable. They both were committed to good communication, and that helped them through the few rough spots they had. They had been friends for so many years before becoming romantic that they knew each other really well. They knew they were very well-matched.

Scott and Diane were married a year after they became involved romantically. After the honeymoon phase was over (and before either of them was diagnosed with ADD), Diane recalled times when she noticed Scott wasn't fully present with her. He might have been physically there, but he wasn't really paying attention mentally or emotionally. He had shifted his focus from her and instead became hyperfocused on his work to the point that he wasn't spending as much time with her.

Problems also surfaced when it came to money management. Scott and Diane both had difficulty managing their money wisely.

They both made a fairly decent living, but neither could figure out where their money went. Try as they might, they were never able to save for a rainy day. Occasionally checks bounced. Twice a month they agonized over paying bills, terrified they would be overdrawn again.

They also both had the ADD habit of interrupting each other and changing topics in the middle of conversations. It might have irritated other people, but since both Scott and Diane had this habit, it didn't bother them when they were speaking to each other.

Scott was the first to be diagnosed with ADD. The diagnosis came when he was in his late thirties. Like Diane, he had always thought something was a little "off" with himself and happened to learn about ADD at a support group for people with Attention Deficit Disorder that his therapist had recommended. "Scales fell from my eyes as I heard other people talk about their ADD and the things they were going through as a result of it," said Scott. With his interest piqued and with support and encouragement from his therapist, Scott sought the help of a psychiatrist who specialized in ADD. He was diagnosed with ADD and immediately started medication, in this case Ritalin. Things started to change for Scott—for the better. The more he learned about ADD, the more he was able to see his own ADD traits. He also started noticing ADD behaviors in Diane. The longer Scott stayed on his medication and was able to see the world around him and his place in it a bit differently, the more clearly he saw Diane, and the more he became convinced that she also had ADD.

Diane, on the other hand, didn't want to have much to do with ADD. Between Scott and all the TV and radio shows about ADD, Diane felt she was being bombarded from all sides. She patiently put up with her husband as he shared information about his new-found hyperfocus, ADD, but Diane did not believe she had it.

The turning point for Diane came when she and Scott attended a conference on ADD in adults. She had agreed to go with him to the conference because they really needed to get away and spend some time together. The more she listened to the talks and seminars, the more she recognized the signs of ADD in herself. All the pieces of her life came together for her. It all finally made sense. After that conference, Diane decided—on her own—to see a physician competent in diagnosing and treating ADD. He formally diagnosed Diane with ADD and began treating her with medications.

In the years since their treatment began, Scott and Diane have continued to build a wonderful life for themselves and their three children. Yes, they both have ADD. But because they have educated themselves about this disorder—and because they're taking medication—they are not living lives that are out of control. In fact, they're probably more in tune with themselves and each other, and more aware when things do start to go wrong, than most non-ADD couples.

For Scott and Diane, ADD is a fact of their lives. It's not necessarily bad or good, it's just a fact that they take into account in understanding their lives and their relationship.

Scott and Diane have developed a set of guidelines that they follow in their home, and some romantic "habits" they both enjoy. These aren't strict rules imposed by an outside source—Scott and Diane have found them helpful in creating a lifestyle that will best nurture their relationship and their children, too. With their permission, I'd like to share some of their beliefs and practices with you now.

1) Don't Argue in the Bedroom.

In Scott and Diane's home, their bedroom is a sacred place. The bedroom is off-limits to fights, frustration, aggravation, and anger. If they're arguing or they're frustrated about something, they talk about it somewhere else. They don't go back into their bedroom until all negative feelings and issues have been dealt with, or until they have come to an agreement with each other to table those conflicts until later. That way they can come back together physically, emotionally, and spiritually and feel connected again. They take a break from the conflict, knowing they can always resolve it in the next day or two. Their bedroom is also completely off-limits to their children, unless the children have specifically been invited in to watch a movie or just to talk. The bedroom is Mom and Dad's special place. If a child wants to come in, they have to knock first and wait at the door until given entrance by Mom or Dad.

2) Love Notes.

Scott and Diane routinely leave love notes for each other. They sneak love notes into each other's wallets or lunch bags. These notes aren't necessarily fancy, and they don't have to be long. A note might just be "I love you" written on a scrap of paper and tucked into a skirt pocket. Sometimes they do leave unexpected greeting cards for each other for no particular occasion. Recently, Scott found a unique little love note tucked into the box of cotton swabs in his bathroom drawer. It was a small rock Diane had collected from the beach with the word "love" beautifully painted on it. Diane not only writes love notes, she writes love rocks! Very creative. Very thoughtful.

3) Date Night.

One night a week is "date night," just for the two of them. The idea of a date night sounds great, until you start to look at the schedules of two working adults and three busy ADD children. That's where the concept of commitment comes in. Scott and Diane are completely committed to their date night. This is a special time for them to be alone and just focus on each other, a time to re-ignite that romantic spark, and they guard this time carefully. They may choose to go to a movie, go to dinner, go for a ride in the country, or send the kids to the baby-sitter's and stay home for a romantic evening of a bubble bath by candlelight. They make certain there is no TV on that night so they can focus on each other and do something that keeps them connected in heart and spirit.

4) Date Weekend.

One weekend a month is "date weekend," just for the two of them. Although this one is often more difficult to schedule, Scott and Diane try to get away one weekend a month without the children. They check into a hotel or go to a bed-and-breakfast. It doesn't even need to be out of town, just away from their daily routine. It's a special time for them to be together and focus just on each other—relaxing, romancing, reconnecting.

5) Love Codes.

In addition to notes on paper, Scott and Diane use their digital pagers to send messages of love. Any couple can develop their own special codes. Scott and Diane use "143" to mean "I love you"—based on the number of letters in each word—or "1432" to mean "I love you, too." If they send "ooooooo" that means lots of hugs, and if they add "911" to the end of all those hugs it means "I want to make love with you." But whatever the particular code is, the person who is receiving the page knows their partner is thinking about them right that minute, even though they are in the middle of a busy day at work.

6) Stay In Touch.

If either of them has to go out of town, they make sure they speak with each other every night. They try not to be apart, but if one of them does have to go out of town for business, they set aside a certain amount of time every night to spend on the phone with each other. That way, they can catch up on each other's day and not feel quite so isolated and separated. Their plan to speak every night says that, even though they may be physically far away, their hearts are not. Their relationship is still a priority.

7) Afternoon Rendezvous.

Sometimes Scott and Diane meet during the day. Occasionally, depending on their work schedules and the children's schedules, they may sneak away and rendezvous for a quiet lunch together. In fact, these brief lunch time getaways are one of Diane's favorite times for them to make love.

8) Educate Yourself About ADD.

By continuing to educate themselves about ADD, Scott and Diane are making a commitment to their relationship. ADD can't get in their way if they understand the disorder and the behaviors it can cause. With their knowledge of Attention Deficit Disorder, they can assess which behaviors are caused by ADD and which aren't. Then, if there's a problem, they can create a solution.

9) Tag-Team Parenting.

When it comes to the children, Scott and Diane take a tag-team approach. Years of experience have taught them that when one parent is upset, things work out best if the other parent makes a special effort to remain calm. This helps their children and also helps their own relationship. With fewer child-related problems, Scott and Diane have fewer negative issues to cloud the little time they do get to spend alone together.

10) Speak Highly of Your Mate.

Scott and Diane consciously make an effort to speak positively about their partner. When Diane does something wonderful at work, Scott tells her how proud he is of her, and vice versa. When talking to colleagues and friends, they purposefully brag about their mate and the things they appreciate about them.

11) Take Your Medication.

Taking medication might not sound very romantic, but when ADD is involved, it helps both partners to nurture each other and the relationship when their brains are working right. Scott and Diane both know that taking their medication as directed will help them be their best for themselves and each other. If Scott or Diane forget to take their medication, they have agreed in advance to table any serious discussion or argument until their medications are back on-board so they can think and process information more productively. That way, they have the best chance to communicate constructively and solve any problems that might come up.

12) Bathe Together.

After a long hard day, relaxing together in the tub is a wonderful way for Scott and Diane to unwind and focus their attention on each other. This isn't something they do every night, but they're always glad when they do make the time for it. It renews their intimacy. These are not just quick baths either. They light candles, dim the lights, and listen to soft music in the background. One of Scott's favorite things is to order Chinese take-out and then bring it home to feed to each other with chopsticks—while in the bathtub together. It's a little crowded and sometimes a little messy eating that way, but it's something they both enjoy together. Besides, if your mate accidentally drops a little food on you while feeding you with chopsticks, creatively cleaning up the mess can be a lot of fun.

13) Send Flowers.

Scott often sends flowers to Diane for no particular reason other than his love for her. And Diane has occasionally been known to reciprocate. It doesn't have to be a big and expensive arrangement from a florist. Sometimes flowers out of their own garden or a single carnation or rose from the floral department at the neighborhood grocery store is all that's needed to get the message of romance and love across.

If you think about this list, you'll see that a lot of what Scott and Diane do in their home is focused on their relationship. Of course, they're also focused on their children and their children's needs. Like any couple, a tremendous amount of time goes into caring for their children. But, unlike many couples—especially couples with ADD, who tend to spend so much time and energy in conflict—Scott and Diane are actively committed to keeping their love and romance alive and well. And in doing that, they are also providing a powerful role model of a positive marriage for their children.

The difference between their relationship now and when they were courting is that their relationship now is much richer. For example, instead of sending flowers because he is hyperfocused on the relationship and the fact that it makes him feel good, Scott might send Diane flowers because he knows she is going through a difficult time that day—either at work or in her personal life. The action might be the same, but the reasoning behind it is very different. Instead of sending the flowers as a way to self-medicate through hyperfocusing on romance, Scott gives a great deal of thought to the ways in which he can best communicate to his wife the tremendous love he feels for her.

Instead of trying to change each other or overlook their differences, Scott and Diane have progressed to the point where they can understand, accept, and even celebrate the differences between them. They watch and learn from each other, they respect each other, and they revel in the commitment and love they have for each other. Scott and Diane utilize the gifts that come with ADD as ways to compensate for the challenges ADD brings to their relationship—to their lives. They have an active love for each other that is always growing. They are supportive when there is pain, loving when there is conflict. They don't do all of these things perfectly. But out of their commitment to each other, to God, and to the institution of marriage itself, they do the best they can each day. Some days they do better, some days they do worse. In spite of their ADD, Scott and Diane continue to grow in their lives and in their love for each other by following the guidelines they have developed over the years for having a wonderfully successful romantic relationship.

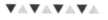

NINE

Help for the Hurting

Scott and Diane, the couple we met in Chapter Eight, really seem to have it all together, don't they? Their relationship has a solid foundation built on a deep love and mutual respect. They understand the ways in which their ADD can negatively affect their relationship, and they have learned how to compensate. They have established mechanisms for dealing with conflict when it arises. And they have made their relationship a priority within the life of their family.

Unfortunately, as we all know, many couples do not have the type of relationship shared by Scott and Diane. Many romantic relationships are built on the shaky foundation of sexual attraction or impulsivity. There is Hollywood's fantasy version of love (that many people confuse with real love) depicted in sitcoms in which relationship problems are humorous and solved in thirty minutes or less. And then there is just hope for a decent relationship, in spite of the fact that the couple may have few, if any, really good relationship skills at all. Then add into a relationship the challenges of ADD. Many people with ADD, or partners of people with ADD, have no clear understanding of either the biological base of ADD or the role it plays in their lives and relationships. Many couples have no positive mechanism for dealing with conflict. And many couples are so busy with work, children, and household chores that they never really make time to nurture the relationship that is at the foundation of their nuclear family.

I think we would all agree that we would prefer to have the type of relationship Scott and Diane share—as opposed to a conflict-driven relationship lacking mutual respect, love, and understanding. And I do believe that if both partners sincerely want to improve their relationship—and both are willing to accept responsibility for the relationship and stop blaming each other—it is certainly possible. On the other hand, there may be times when it's best to call it quits.

But how do you know when it's really time to get some professional help for your relationship? And how do you know if it's time to end the relationship? Let's take a look.

Unfortunately, most people wait until it's too late before they finally start seeking help for their troubled relationship. They keep thinking and hoping that things will get better, but things don't. I'd like to borrow the definition of insanity as defined by Alcoholics Anonymous to describe this kind of situation. Insanity is when we keep doing the same things over and over again and each time expect different results. If you don't change what you are doing, the results of your actions will continue to be the same—in this case, futile.

If you and your mate are having a problem and you see the same problem surface numerous times, that's probably an indication that you need to do something different. If you can't figure out what it is you need to do differently, seek some outside help. If you knew how to change on your own, you would probably do it. But it's insane to keep making the same mistakes over and over. A qualified marriage and family therapist who knows a lot about ADD can offer insights and tools for making a relationship better. Apply what you learn from the therapist and find new ways—more productive ways—to make your relationship work. Don't wait until the *Titanic* is three feet under water before you sound the alarm and start taking precautions to keep the ship from sinking. By then, it's too late.

How do you know whether or not you need help? And will you actually get the help you need?

Your ability to answer those questions is somewhat determined by the relationship you witnessed firsthand growing up—your parents' marriage. Did your parents go through difficult times in their own marriage? Did they seek counseling or other forms of help? Did they work hard to overcome any difficulties they might have had? Did they stay together? Did they get divorced?

What you saw as a child influences your views of your own relationship now.

For example, some of us grew up with parents who took their marriage vows literally and decided that divorce would never be an option. These people stay married until one of them dies, regardless of whether or not they have a good relationship. In good times, these couples enjoy the security of their marriage. In bad times, they hang in there no matter what. Some couples in this situation are able to work things through, get past the bad times, and continue on in an improved marriage. Others spend their entire married lives in miserable, emotionally void relationships—because they are committed to staying married at all costs, but lack the tools and skills needed to make their relationship a positive and healthy one.

Others grew up with divorced parents. This type of couple—particularly if both the husband and wife were children of divorce— might be more likely to consider divorce as an option for themselves. And if ADD is involved, people are just as likely to divorce on impulse as they were to get married on impulse, even if that decision isn't really in their best long-term interest.

On the other hand, children of divorce are sometimes even more committed to making their relationship work, particularly if they have children. They've experienced firsthand the complex emotional trauma that divorce causes for children. It just depends on the specific personalities involved.

In any case, a couple's concept of marriage, as influenced by childhood experiences, can have a tremendous impact, one way or the other, on the longevity of the relationship.

Of the research I've seen and heard about marriage and what I have learned from all the couples I have worked with professionally over the years, I've come to believe that most couples tend to bail out of the relationship way too early, before they've really done the work necessary to create a solid relationship. They end up repeating the same mistakes with their next partner and then their next and so on.

A good relationship takes work.

A friend of mine who is a family physician often sees patients who are going through marital problems. He has a standard response when his patients begin to share their frustration and pain. "Relationships are not easy." The really successful marriages, like Scott and Diane's, are relationships in which both partners are willing to work for and invest in their marriage. Certainly, they have difficult times when conflicts seem insurmountable—all relationships go through that to some degree or another—but they hang in there and keep working on it. They keep growing and learning. They don't abandon ship when the seas get rough. They may feel like abandoning ship sometimes, but they stay on course. And when necessary, they weather the storms together, knowing that the sun *will* shine again, that there *will* be calm seas again.

There is a lot to be said about the ADD style of stick-to-itiveness that adds to the success of Scott and Diane's marriage. If there are problems, they don't wait until it's too late to repair the relationship.

Often, by the time a couple comes in for therapy, their marriage is in very serious trouble. Their pain becomes so great that they finally push past their shame of "having to go to therapy" and show up emotionally battered and bruised on the therapist's doorstep expecting the therapist to work an instant miracle. This is one of the biggest frustrations for therapists. With barely a breath of life left in the relationship, the couple wants a quick fix to take away all the pain and breathe life back into something that has been dying from neglect or abuse for far too long. And insurance companies sometimes cover three to six visits and then no more. The financial pressure of having to pay out of pocket for treatment that is taking too long to present a miracle, plus the commitment to keep coming back each week for several weeks without seeing an immediate response, is sometimes too much stress for one or both partners and they abandon ship.

If they had only come in sooner, there would have been a much greater opportunity to help them work through their problems, and a much greater chance of repairing the relationship. The longer people stay in the same problem-causing behaviors, the more difficult it is to change those behaviors.

In addition to seeking marriage therapy as soon as you see problems arise and repeat, it may become necessary to take some time off from the intensity of the relationship. Don't be afraid to take a break if you need it. Cool off. Stay with a friend for a few days. Rent a hotel room for a week and sort out your thoughts, feelings, and desires in solitude. Sometimes just being away from each other for a day or so helps individuals in the relationship to regroup and regain perspective, to see what's going on and how and where they may need to make changes in their recipe for a fabulous relationship. This brief time apart can often be a positive experience that can help in problem-solving when the two partners come back together again.

See if you can let it be okay for one or both of you to create some *temporary* distance, to step away from the conflicts and reflect upon the love, goals, and dreams the two of you started with. Sometimes the best way to refocus your perspective is to remove yourself from the situation for a short period of time. In the quietness of that retreat, you can reassess and rediscover who you are, who your partner is, and what it is that you want but are not getting. You can then share this information with your partner.

If you choose to invest in the future of your relationship by going to therapy, you need to see a therapist that both of you can feel good about—a therapist who is *the therapist for the relationship* (the actual patient), not for each individual partner. Find a therapist who knows ADD inside and out, and seek their help and guidance to find healing for the *relationship*.

Therapy should never be a situation in which the first partner drags the second partner into therapy with the intent of having the therapist ridicule and blame the second partner as the cause of all the problems in the relationship. That wouldn't be therapy. That would be abuse. Relationship therapy is designed to help each partner see what strengths and weaknesses they each bring to the relationship and how to compensate for the weaknesses by capitalizing on the strengths. It's about becoming a team.

There are great therapists and not-so-great therapists, just like there are great plumbers and not-so-great plumbers. So shop for a therapist wisely. Interview several therapists just as you would if you were shopping for a new painter, lawyer, or doctor. Remember, a therapist is not God. A therapist is simply a professional whom you are hiring to provide you with a specific service. So make sure you and your partner are both comfortable with a therapist before you hire that person. You'll need to feel a sense of mutual trust—never a condescending attitude—so you'll be able to be honest and progress toward your goals. Make sure you understand clearly the mechanics of the relationship—fees, appointment scheduling, etc. Remember, you are the consumer, and therapy is the product you are purchasing. So do your research.

Most importantly, don't wait too long to get the help you need. Get help while the problems are easier to resolve. It might not sound appealing at this moment, but I suggest you embrace your pain as your friend, because your pain is there for a reason. It's there to tell you that something needs to change—most likely something inside of you.

Chapter Ten, "The Sweetheart Approach," will provide you with some positive ways to move forward in change. It provides a strong foundation from which to build a better relationship and attitudes that can help you right now in working through the problems you may currently be facing. If you need to, put a bookmark here and skip forward for a quick grasp of that encouragement. But remember to come back and finish this chapter. There may be some very important information here that you need.

We've talked about the importance of getting into therapy when things start getting rough in general. Now we're going to look at some very specific "land mines" to watch out for and what to do if and when these problems come your way.

Verbal and Emotional Abuse

We hear a lot in the media about physical and sexual abuse. We'll be covering those subjects too, but first let's look at some other forms of abuse that leave bruises and scars of a different nature— bruises and scars to the heart and soul of a person through verbal and emotional abuse. Although there may not be any visible cuts and bruises, the injuries are still very real and very present.

Verbal abuse is verbally overpowering your partner. Yelling at them. Threatening them. Barraging them with vocal assaults. Terrifying them through verbal bravado. It is about control and manipulation through demanding and demeaning commands. It is not about loving them. It is not about encouraging them. It only serves one purpose: to control by power and force. It only has one result: damage. Damage to the person on the receiving end of the abuse and damage to the relationship.

Verbal and emotional abuse are every bit as painful and traumatic as any kind of physical abuse. Perhaps the most common aspect of abuse in romantic relationships associated with ADD are emotional and verbal abuse. These forms of abuse can often take place without the ADD person even knowing they're doing it. Cutting words delivered impulsively. Promises not fulfilled. Flash anger. All of these things contribute daily to the demise of the relationship. Slowly, but continuously, the strength of the relationship is chipped away by these kinds of unchecked and untreated ADD behaviors. Plus, there is also the verbal and emotional abuse the non-ADD partner can inflict out of their frustrations with the ADD behaviors. Although each partner might not be physically assaulting the other, it takes an emotional (and physical) toll to hear over and over again: "You're so stupid! What's wrong with you? You always screw things up. You're never going to amount to anything!" Unfortunately, all too often, partners who suffer from this type of abuse begin to believe these things about themselves. Their self-esteem drops to all-time lows, and while in a state of emotional upheaval they regress to their lowest level of functioning (a natural human response). They move into a fight-or-flight survival mode. Their basic instinct at that point is not about having a wonderful relationship, it is to "kill or be killed."

So at a time in the relationship when they need relationship skills the most, the individual is hard-pressed to access those skills because they are in survival mode. At that point, the problems in the relationship become compounded. When we are in survival mode, our focus is on protecting ourselves rather than learning and growing. It is a natural human response, but one that is not necessarily going to help much in working through the problems they're having in their relationship. People need to feel safe if they are to self-actualize and grow. It is difficult to feel safe when you and your partner are throwing rocks at each other, whether the rocks are cutting words and demeaning behaviors or real rocks.

Think of a seven-year-old child in a classroom trying to learn. If it's too noisy in the classroom—or if the child has learning disabilities—it's going to be more difficult for him to learn. But if you then add a large, mean, overpowering teacher standing next to the child, embarrassing him in front of his friends, he won't be able to concentrate and get his math done . . . chances are, he'll just freeze up and do nothing. Even if the child works on his class assignment at that moment, it will most likely be full of mistakes. Why? The child is terrified. His brain and body leave math and lock into fear. The child is afraid of what could happen to him. Not the best way to learn math, or any subject, for that matter.

So the child's performance worsens, as does his self-esteem. He develops phobias of both school and math and cries each morning as his parents force him to return to a place of torture each day. The child develops an automatic fear response to anything that seems similar in any way, shape, or form to the horrifying experiences at school. Terrified, he remains in a heightened state of hyper-vigilance and fear, making it most difficult to learn.

Verbal and emotional abuse cause that same kind of response in adults when the perpetrator moves out of a peer position in the relationship and forcefully maneuvers himself into a perceived position of authority, successfully manipulating his partner into a place of submission. She regresses to a childhood ego state and for all intents and purposes becomes the terrified child in the example above. Since the perpetrator is perceived to have all the authority, she feels trapped. Although she wants to leave, she's often unable to without professional help from a therapist or women's support group.

Verbal and emotional abuse are two major tools that have been used in wartime to try to persuade the enemy into submission. This was certainly true in World War II when Tokyo Rose broadcast erroneous and seductive messages to our troops indicating and intimating that they should give up. Whether it's war with other countries or war with our spouse, verbal and emotional abuse are powerful "brainwashing" tools in the arsenal of psychological warfare. Spouses at war with each other is not a romantic or loving situation.

Emotional abuse can be both overt and covert. Overt emotional abuse is about belittling someone. Through verbal assaults, manipulating them to feel less than adequate. Putting down someone either through direct accusations or indirectly through off-handed comments that destroy their spirit. It is about psychologically manipulating someone into a place of submission and servitude.

Emotional abuse robs the attacked of their self-esteem, self-concept, and freedom to be. And most often this is done through verbal attacks that cut to the very core of the person, with the intent to conquer and destroy them. Then they are no longer a threat to the attacker. The attacker does not have to face the sheer terror of having to see themselves as dysfunctional. Of needing to change. Of being wrong.

The other most common versions of emotional abuse are done covertly. Playing mind games. Emotionally and mentally jerking their partner around until they don't know which end is up. This type of abuse might include stalking their lover. It may mean making phone calls in the middle of the night to them, but never saying a thing and just hanging up—with the purpose of scaring them. It may mean threatening to physically harm them, although the abuser may never actually become physical. The threat is the abuse. The tactic is to scare in order to control. The perpetrator may punch walls or throw things as ways to reinforce what could happen if they don't get their way. Mind you, this is very different from someone who may throw something or punch walls because they are so frustrated and don't know how to deal with their anger in appropriate ways. But it should also be noted that these two intentions—terrorism and frustration—are not necessarily mutually exclusive.

Covert emotional abuse might include choosing not to talk to their partner for days on end as a way to punish or manipulate them into submission. It may mean using sexual intimacy—or the lack thereof—as a way to control. There are many ways to covertly manipulate someone into submission through emotional abuse.

If you are in a relationship that involves emotional abuse, whether that abuse is overt or covert, you need the help of a therapist to learn how to better take care of yourself. Do everything it takes to get into therapy now.

Emotional and Sexual Affairs—The Abuse of Trust

Defining or identifying an emotional affair can be difficult at times because it has to do with one's intentions. Emotional affairs occur when a spouse becomes involved in an emotionally intimate relationship in which physical sexual activity has not taken place. If left unchecked, that emotional intimacy often leads to sexual intimacy. So although the behaviors associated with an emotional affair can look quite harmless to begin with—"we were just talking"—they can lead to disaster down the road.

People with ADD or spouses of people with ADD can fall prey to this kind of affair very easily. They look for a sympathetic shoulder to cry on when upset with their spouse—someone who will listen and understand without interrupting, who is more stimulating at the moment, who "needs" me more than my spouse needs me.

The more time spent with such an outsider, the less time spent intimately sharing with one's spouse.

Trust and intimacy are two of the major ingredients in the glue that binds two people together. The more time spent bonding with the outsider, the more likely the marriage will eventually flounder and fail. Emotional intimacy can certainly lead to sexual affairs, which assuredly will damage their relationship even further. But emotional intimacy can also lead to a situation in which an adult partner is spending more time bonding intimately—emotionally—with their children than they are with their spouse. Although we don't talk a lot about emotional affairs and excessive emotional bonding with one's children, it happens a lot. These are not benign behaviors. They need to be taken very seriously and seen for what they are: breaches of trust and confidence in the relationship.

Most often, emotional affairs begin due to a breakdown in communication. So go back and read the chapter on communication skills and get into therapy to learn how to communicate better. Avoid the trap of "innocent" little get-togethers that often lead to sexual affairs and the eventual demise of the relationship. This is not to say that you can't have friends of the opposite sex, or that you shouldn't be close to your children. It means that when emotional intimacy with someone other than your partner is for the purpose of avoiding intimacy with your partner, it's a breeding ground for infections which may contaminate and possibly even kill the relationship.

Sexual affairs are much easier to define than emotional affairs. Sexual affairs are evidenced by any sexual activity with someone other than one's spouse. This includes behaviors ranging from holding hands, kissing, or fondling to sexual intercourse—vaginally, orally, or otherwise.

If you or your partner are having a sexual affair in addition to the other problems already in your relationship, you both need to get help fast. Sexual affairs are the biggest, most deadly threats to the life and quality of any romantic relationship. If you are the one having the affair, a therapist could help you discover the reasons behind your affair and how it is affecting the dynamics between you and your partner—and for that matter, your life in general. If your partner is the one having the affair, a therapist could help you better understand and deal with your own feelings as you come to grips with your partner's behavior.

Sometimes spouses are aware that their partner is having an affair and still choose to stay in the relationship. Your life is probably not overtly threatened in this situation. However, if your partner is not practicing safe sex, your life is certainly threatened covertly due to the epidemic of AIDS. If you decide to stay in this type of relationship, for whatever reasons you may have, you *must* practice safe sex with your partner. AIDS is no respecter of class, culture, money, religion, or gender. Having sex with a spouse who is having extramarital sexual affairs means you are also having sex with the person (or the people) they are having sex with—and the people that *they* had sex with. You can't know if they are practicing safe sex, so it's up to you to make certain that *you* practice safe sex with your partner.

For more information about how to practice safe sex, call your local county department of health. You can make an anonymous phone call. They will never know who you are unless you tell them. Most agency personnel are very careful not to judge or shame people who call for information. They know that we as a culture are very skittish when it comes to talking about sex in the first place. Their only desire is to do whatever they can to help stop the spread of AIDS and to save lives—possibly yours.

If you or your partner are having an affair, you both need to be in therapy—individual therapy *and* couples therapy. There are a lot of dynamics and issues to work through when sexual affairs are happening or have taken place. You will both need to work together with a qualified couples therapist to try to work through these issues. This therapist must also be someone who really understands ADD and the issues and mechanisms that trigger affairs.

Should you divorce your partner for having a sexual affair? You'll need to decide that for yourself. Certainly, there are relationships that have weathered the stormy seas created in the wake of sexual affairs and have come through those storms only to have a much better and stronger relationship than they ever had before. Marriages in which the couple develops a stronger sense of love and connectedness through all the hard work they had to go through to save the marriage. Should you give up the ship? Only you can say.

Just as there are plenty of relationships that have survived those storms, there are just as many—probably more—that did not survive because of an affair. Personal values, religious beliefs, ego strength, and social pressure are just some of the factors that go into deciding whether to stay in or leave a relationship tainted by a sexual affair. Talk with your pastor, priest, or rabbi. Talk with your therapist. Talk with friends you can trust. Talk with your spouse. But ultimately, it is you who will have to decide what to do.

There may be several reasons why the affair began in the first place. It might be partly due to ADD impulsivity. It may be that there were other problems in the relationship to begin with and the affair is only the tip of that iceberg. Whatever the reasons, if you decide you still want the relationship, get some help sorting out all of the different thoughts and feelings that come into play when there has been a sexual indiscretion. Therapy can help. But so many people look to therapy as a way to get someone else to "beat up" their spouse for them. If you envision dragging your partner into therapy and having the therapist berate them for their behavior and verbally beat them into submission, then you don't really understand the goal of therapy. The goal of couples therapy should be to help individuals examine and improve their relationships, not to abuse your partner (in retaliation) for his or her inappropriate behavior.

As we saw in Chapter Six, sometimes people can be addicted to sex—or the adrenaline and endorphin rush that comes from the thrill and excitement of sex with a different partner. They can use that rush to self-medicate their ADD. And that behavior can obviously become a very serious problem in their relationship.

Another sign of sexual addiction is a person who continues to have affairs, even though he or she really wants to stop that behavior but just can't seem to. If you or your partner has this problem, there is a twelve-step program that addresses this issue. The name of the group is Sex and Love Addicts Anonymous (SLAA). Because of the shame associated with sexual addiction, SLAA groups can be a little hard to find. And chances are it's easier to find a local group in a larger city. Ask your therapist for a referral or call the SLAA national headquarters at (617) 332-1845 to find a chapter in your area.

Physical Abuse

Perhaps the most serious situation, and the one that clearly needs the most immediate action and the most intense help, is a relationship that involves physical abuse.

When we hear the term "physical abuse," we usually think of the images the media has brought to our attention so often. And we may remember the deadly ramifications of victims who did not take the warning signs of this form of abuse seriously enough. We've all heard horror stories of husbands who stalk, emotionally torture, and sometimes even hunt down and kill their ex-wives. Stories of women who are afraid to leave their home—or go home—because they are emotionally isolated and physically beaten by their husbands.

If you're in an abusive relationship—especially if physical abuse is involved—*you must get yourself physically out of that relationship now.*

I really cannot emphasize this enough. If you're in an abusive relationship—*get out now.*

I know this advice is much easier to give than to take. I know that if you are in an abusive relationship, there often seem to be 100 reasons not to leave. You love your partner. He said he would never do it again. Or she only acts like this when she's drunk, and she promised she'll never drink again. You can't imagine living on your own, especially if you have children. You're simply afraid to leave—afraid he'll find you and the abuse will be even worse. Or you really love your partner and believe you can help her get over this type of sadistic behavior.

But no matter what your reasons are for not leaving, you must remember this one crucial point: If you are alive, you can always go back to the relationship to try to solve your problems another day. If you are not alive, you will never, ever have the chance to make that choice. When it comes down to the bottom line, it's really that simple.

Think about this. If you're in an abusive relationship and are choosing to stay in that relationship, something is wrong. *You* have a problem and you need to get help for it. If for whatever reason you are unable to remove yourself from a potentially harmful situation, the first thing you need to do is to see a mental health professional—a psychiatrist, psychologist, or family therapist—for some help. A competent therapist will know how to help you, even if it's just to make referrals to other professionals who would know how to help you. You've got to start somewhere. Do whatever it takes to get out without getting hurt and without trying to retaliate against your partner. It doesn't necessarily mean that you will never be together with your partner again. If you both really do love each other, through intense psychotherapy and other treatment protocols the two of you may be able to get back together again and recreate the relationship you both had dreams for in the first place. But again, there is no chance of that happening if the two of you continue to stay together, refuse to get help, and end up killing each other.

Maybe you're not the one suffering the abuse. Maybe you're the abuser. Or maybe you've never hit another person, but you feel so much anger inside, you just feel like you could put your hand through the wall any minute. If you're in any of these situations, you need to see a psychiatrist to get the medical help you need to help treat your rage.

Let's be clear about something. When we hear "you need to see a psychiatrist," we often interpret that as a put-down. "What are you telling me? Are you telling me that I'm crazy? Are you telling me that I'm hopeless and need to be put away?" No. And I wish that very old stereotypical view of mental health professionals would disappear. But if you're raging, you have a problem and you need to get help for it.

If your tooth were hurting, you'd visit a dentist. If you couldn't see well, you'd visit an eye doctor. But since the pain you're experiencing is in the area of emotions, particularly despair or anger, you need to visit a psychiatrist. Psychiatrists have the training and ability to look at your symptoms and correlate them with metabolic patterns in your brain that heavily influence how you act and react to other people and your environment. Often, through medical interventions, much of the rage may go away by itself. It's often really that simple—and that important.

I would also suggest that you pick up a copy of my book called *Anger, Rage and Hope*. In that book, you'll find information about anger, and anger management, as well as exercises you can do on a daily basis to help you better manage your anger.

Managing anger is extremely important, both to protect your partner from any physical violence your anger might lead to, and for your own mental, emotional, and even physical health. In most major cities, there are self-help groups that deal solely with anger management. Usually the court system refers offenders to these kinds of groups. The court should be able to give you names and phone numbers of a local group you can get involved with. But whatever approach you take, take action now before someone gets hurt. It's up to you. Do whatever it takes and get the help you need now.

Despair

Sometimes people who are trying hard to make a relationship work get so frustrated and discouraged that they start feeling helpless, hopeless, and sometimes, even suicidal. If you're having any of those kinds of feelings, you need to get to a physician, preferably a psychiatrist, as soon as possible. These three things are often symptoms of major depression and need to be taken seriously. Mental health, like any health issue, needs to be treated by a qualified physician. During stressful times we need all the mental and emotional strength we can garner in order to survive and thrive. There are many ways to approach treatment. Medication prescribed by a physician is often the way to go. But medication is not the only way to treat depression.

In addition to medication—but not necessarily instead of medication—I recommend therapy. That way, you can work with someone to understand what's going on in your life and why. And that therapist will have resources of groups and individuals who can help you deal with and/or leave your abusive situation, whether it's a battered-spouse support group, a women's shelter, or some other type of safe house.

In addition to medication prescribed by a psychiatrist, and in addition to therapy, you need to also be working a twelve-step program. In a twelve-step program, you'll find people just like you who have been through what you're going through right now, people who really do know how you feel. These people will be able to give you a kind of support that no one else can give. They've been there. And they know.

At a good twelve-step meeting there are no judgments placed on you about anything. It's a place where you can be safe to listen and learn. A safe place where you're allowed to just be yourself so that you might discover who you really are.

Most importantly, when you find the right group, you will begin to feel less alone. A sense of being alone with your problems—a sense of separation from the rest of your family and community—is one of the most difficult and damaging feelings for people to deal with. And abusers often try to seclude their victims from the outside world so they have no support to help them stay strong and individual. So it's vital to your safety and recovery that you go to meetings regularly.

But here's the truth, and don't ever forget it: Whatever it is you're going through, no matter how bad it really is, there are thousands of other people, just like you, facing similar problems. And through twelve-step programs, you can connect with those kindred spirits.

Depending on where you live, there may be many different types of twelve-step programs available to you. The primary organization to consider is called Codependents Anonymous (CoDA). CoDA is a twelve-step program created especially for people who are having problems in their relationships. You may be able to find CoDA listed in the white pages of your local phone book. Or you can call their national headquarters in Phoenix at (602) 277-7991, and that office will be able to tell you where the closest meetings are taking place. If you don't have any CoDA meetings in your local area, try attending a meeting of another twelve-step program, such as Al-Anon, a support group for people in relationships with alcoholics. Whatever issue the group addresses will be helpful for you.

You can find help and healing by working the twelve-step with other people in recovery, going to therapy regularly, and taking medication provided by a qualified physician. Now that you have this information, it's up to you to take whatever actions necessary to stay safe and alive so you and your partner can work through the relationship challenges you presently face. If you're ever fearful for your life or safety, call 9-1-1 to get help immediately. Leave the relationship if you need to. Stay in the relationship if you need to stay. But for goodness' sake, stop the insanity of doing the same things over and over again, each time expecting different results. If nothing changes, nothing changes.

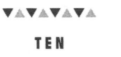

TEN

The Sweetheart Approach

In working with hundreds of ADD couples, I've identified ten basic concepts that can be used to enhance relationships—concepts that can form a foundation for the kind of relationship you've always wanted. I'd like to share them with you now. Each is a simple truth. Each is incredibly important. And to help you remember them, each letter of the word *Sweetheart* stands for one of the concepts. Hence, "The Sweetheart Approach." Let's get started.

The first letter in Sweetheart is "S", which stands for STRUC-TURE. One of the best tools for dealing with ADD is structure. Structure gives the easily distracted person something to hang onto when the tendency is to fly off to another thought or activity. For example, you and your partner sit down and decide together to scrimp and save this year so you can take your dream vacation—a Mediterranean cruise—next year. You've just created structure—you have a plan. That wasn't so hard, was it? Where most people have problems is when they don't adhere to the plan they have already set up for themselves. Why? A hallmark of ADD is being easily distracted. Sure, you've got the *plan* to scrimp and save for that dream vacation, but then comes this great deal on a new sports car or the holiday sales which gobble up your money (and your plan) and leave you with another dreary campout in your own backyard instead of sailing the *Love Boat* on a romantic Mediterranean cruise.

When you've agreed to a plan, there is an element of commitment, and that commitment is where the real structure comes into play. Structure is a way to anchor yourself to reliability. When we're so easily distracted by other "stuff," we need structure to keep us from flying off to the next stimulating idea or activity.

"One minute we have plans to go to the movies, the next, he's changed his mind and now wants to go fishing with his friends! I can't keep up with him and I can't trust anything he says. This is driving me crazy!"

How often have you said, felt, or heard something similar to this? Structure will help keep this kind of scatteredness to a minimum and will lessen the stress it creates in a relationship.

I realize that some people are terrified of writing down goals (structure). I know, because I am one of those people. But I also know that having a plan and following that plan is incredibly powerful.

It is of utmost importance that the two of you create your plan together. Engineer it in such a way that you both get your needs met. To borrow a slogan from my friends in recovery, it's a matter of first having a plan and then working that plan. I add to that: Have a plan and work that plan *regardless of how you feel*. This kind of structure will help you build the foundation for a better, more satisfying relationship, one in which both of you will have your needs met. If you don't get your needs met in appropriate ways, you will find ways of getting them met inappropriately—that's just human nature. But that's not going to help the relationship.

Some people with ADD have difficulty with the idea of structure at first, feeling that they're going to lose their freedom to be who they are—free and spontaneous. In fact, a friend of mine who has ADD told me that he was terrified of losing his spontaneity by having to work things through a planned system, by having to adhere to structure. Of course we're resistant to structure. We're so used to being so easily distracted that to have to stick to something—to have to stay on task—literally can cause some of us to feel extremely anxious and very uncomfortable.

People without ADD may have a difficult time understanding that some of us have a tremendous amount of anxiety about structure. Our fear is that it will restrict our natural tendency to fly from one thing to another. It literally can feel to us what it must feel like for a wild bird to be tethered and unable to fly. And yet, if we are to succeed in creating a fabulous romantic relationship, one that can last a lifetime, we must learn how to embrace structure.

"It's hard!" I've heard those words many times over the years, and what I tell people is, "No, it's not. It's just new." Anything that is new is going to seem hard at first. You didn't learn to walk in one day, it took a lot of practice. And when you were learning to walk, what made it easier, what was encouraging, was all the cheering you got from the sidelines, by your parents. It didn't matter if you wobbled with unsteady legs, or fell on your keister and got right back up to try walking again, they were there for you. With encouragement and with persistence, you eventually learned to walk. And now you do it quite well without even thinking about it.

Structure does take some getting used to, but after you've learned how to be comfortable with it, you can also learn how to run with it. When you and your mate have co-engineered structure and adhere to it, that gives you the ability to run together, side by side. And that's why you got together in the first place, wasn't it—so you could go through life together?

The kind of structure we're talking about needs two basic components. It needs to be flexible enough to adjust for opportunities and diversity, yet rigid enough to keep you on track so you are not easily swayed (distracted) to the left or to the right when you need to be going straight ahead. This is a delicate balance that may take some time for both partners to learn how to engineer together. But then, you've got time, right? Remember, "Till death do us part."

"Till death do us part? That may come sooner than he thinks! Just because I have ADD, he tries to control every move I make! I don't feel I can even go soak in the tub after work without him pointing out the tasks I haven't finished yet. Give me a break!"

Remember, structure needs to be engineered by both of you. If one partner is trying to impose structure on the other partner, it will feel like a prison, like one partner has locked the other partner to a ball and chain—and how many times have we heard that derogatory phrase in relation to a mate? One person trying to enforce structure will not help the relationship at all.

To *choose* to let go of something for the sake of the relationship is very different from having it taken away. Make sure you're both winners when you develop your structure. Do it together.

Those couples who practice putting structure into their lives and into their romance—even though it may be uncomfortable at first—find that, after a while, it becomes something they embrace. This is partly due to the fact that, once the structure *is* in place, they can let go of having to keep a constant watch on what they're supposed to do or not do. Those decisions have already been mapped out in their plan. When people learn to fall back and rely on structure, it actually allows them to free their minds, which opens other doors for creativity. Yes! The right kind of structure can ultimately free you.

You can be free from having to worry about making impulsive, last-minute decisions because you and your partner already have a plan in place. A plan that will help you both stay on track with your agreed-upon goals—goals that will satisfy both of your needs. The structure you have dreaded for so long may be the very thing you have needed to set yourself free and finally take that Mediterranean cruise, instead of vacationing in the backyard and wondering what happened to your dream vacation.

Let's move on to "W", which stands for WELCOME. Welcome the differences between the two of you. Being different from each other is partly why you chose each other in the first place. People have different points of view. It's important that we learn to embrace not only our own point of view but also our partner's point of view. When you feel as if your partner is doing something or has an opinion that you think is stupid, you might want to take a look and see where you are stuck in *your* thinking. Try to see what your partner's point of view is and why it makes sense to *them*. Try to see things from *their* perspective. After all, we *all* have blind sides. When you're in opposition to your partner's thoughts or beliefs, stop for a moment. Remember the Sweetheart Approach. Welcome the differences. Take a moment to look, really look, at what they are seeing. It's very possible that they might have a handle on something you can't because your life experiences are limiting you in this particular area. It just may be that their point of view is the one that can save you from disaster.

"She never listens to what I have to say! She always has to be right, even when she's wrong. It's like what I have to say doesn't even matter."

Is this your experience—or is it what your partner feels after numerous interactions in which you don't embrace the differences between the two of you? That whole attitude, which is often pervasive in ADD folks, not only can cause major disruption to the relationship, it can also cause serious damage to your partner's self-esteem. That doesn't sound like loving behavior, does it?

Regardless of whether it is you or your partner who has the "right" point of view, if you don't learn to welcome the differences and embrace each other's point of view, you may be taking a trip from the altar to the attorney's office in relatively short order.

I'm not saying that you have to give up your own point of view. What I'm saying is that it's important that you welcome the differences. See if maybe there is something you're missing in your partner's point of view, see if that information can help both of you to make a better decision together.

As the two of you learn to welcome and embrace the differences in each other, there are sure to be conflicts along the way. By welcoming the differences and showing respect for your partner and their point of view, you may be able to even learn how to welcome conflict.

Welcome conflict? Yes. Not necessarily argue and bicker, but welcome divergent ideas and use those ideas in a synergistic way to create a greater and better idea than you as an individual could have come up with on your own. That's the beauty of synergism. When we learn how to use conflict this way, it helps the relationship and helps the partners get more of what they want in life. And since people with ADD are hooked on stimulation, it creates a lot of stimulation, but in a healthy way.

You can both learn to use conflict as a way to create closeness. Learn to see the *conflict* as the problem that needs to be solved, not your *partner*. Be a team. As a team, work together to solve the problem in a way that is mutually satisfying for both of you. You will find this technique is very easy with just a little practice.

The next letter in Sweetheart is the letter "E", which stands for ENCOURAGE. Learn to encourage each other. Relationships are hard enough to begin with. Add ADD and it really gets interesting. Use structure to remind yourself to say encouraging things to each other every day. If the person with ADD was able to stay more focused or was less impulsive, acknowledge that. It's a major accomplishment. Celebrate it. And if the non-ADD partner is able to let go and laugh about something instead of criticizing their ADD partner, acknowledge them!

The world can be a really rough place at times, and you both need each other for encouragement. Structure that into your lives so that it's always present.

"It's amazing! All she said to me was she was proud of me for trying. I could see it in her eyes. She meant it. That's all I needed to hear. I felt closer to her than I have in a long time and that felt really good."

Encouragement is such an important part of life that a very famous psychiatrist named Alfred Adler concluded that satisfaction and fulfillment in life are largely a result of encouragement. If a person is discouraged, the discouragement will take a major toll on their emotional and mental well-being. In fact, one of Adler's basic tenets was that mental illness has at its root the disease of discouragement. If that's the case, we all need a little encouragement. In fact, we probably need a lot of encouragement.

When you see your partner doing something that is "right" or more effective or more nurturing or more gentle, encourage them. Celebrate them. Acknowledge them for their accomplishment. When it's your turn to be on the receiving end of the encouraging, stop for a moment. Listen—really listen—to your partner's acknowledgment of *you*. Take it into your heart and hold it there for more than just a fleeting moment. Take hold of that kindness and let it be the talisman that carries you safely on your journey through the rest of the day.

As you practice encouraging each other, you each become what I call a "safe person." A safe person is someone who will listen without judgment or without trying to fix the problem or the other person. They are more ready to accept and understand than to judge or reprimand. They are willing to be with you in your feelings rather than tell you that you should feel something else. They are someone who will say—possibly even through silence: "I'm still with you—all the way."

Practice encouragement. Make certain you both have this most important life force flowing through your relationship.

We're up to the fourth letter in Sweetheart, which is another "E". This time, it stands for EASY DOES IT. Learning new ways of interacting with each other when ADD is involved can be a lot of work. Be gentle with each other. If things get to be too hectic, take some time out. If you get stuck in an argument, agree to take a break and go to a movie (maybe even together). Do something to change the focus. If all you see is frustration or aggravation, choose to look at something more uplifting for a while.

A couple thousand years ago a very wise man recognized this when he wrote the words, "Dwell on those things that are good and pure." You can always return to the conflict later if you need to. Give yourself a break. Allow yourself time to work through and process these things. Give yourself and your partner the space to be imperfect—the grace to be human. If you don't know how to handle a situation any better than you do right now, let it be. Use that information to guide you and direct you to learning and using new skills that *will* help your relationship. If you discover you don't have the skills or the tools to handle the conflicts, find out where you can get them. See a therapist. Go to a support group. Use your awareness of your weaknesses as the inspiration to learn new skills. Don't use your insight as a weapon to batter yourself or your partner emotionally.

Most decisions do not have to be made in an instant. Most conflicts do not have to be resolved in an instant. So be gentle, and take it easy on yourself and each other. And when necessary, take a break.

When you do, it is helpful to mutually agree to the break. One of you may have to take the break on your own initiative, but if possible see if you can agree together to take a "time-out." Sometimes a time-out is all that's needed to let go of the issue. Sometimes it's not. Sometimes things need to be discussed further in order to resolve a conflict. If more time is needed, take the break but also agree to get back together at a later time to finish the process. This will give each of you a chance to think about the conflict, your needs, and your partner's needs. It will also give you a chance to incorporate what your partner has been saying. When you've both had a chance to cool down a little, you can come back together later to resolve the conflict.

Those of us with ADD can be very impatient. If there's a conflict, we want it solved now. If there's an answer that needs to be agreed upon, we want that agreement made now. We need to learn how to let go, which can be very hard to do. Once again, that's when we return to the Sweetheart Approach, and use the letter "E" to remind us: easy does it. It doesn't have to be decided right now. Let go of it for awhile. It's possible to *learn* how to do this. Medication makes the learning process a lot easier. In the meantime, whether you are on medication or not, the idea of "easy does it" is still important and something that can be learned and utilized effectively.

The letter "T" in the word Sweetheart stands for TRUST—both trusting and being trustworthy. If the two of you are going to work together as a team in dealing with ADD and learning how to have the wonderful relationship you have always dreamed of, you need trust.

"I can't trust anything he says! I've had enough disappointments for a lifetime!"

Does this sound familiar? Have you said these very words or something similar, or have you been on the receiving end of this kind of comment? This is an example of trust being undermined in the relationship. It's a road sign pointing to greater pain and frustration if something is not done soon to restore trust to the relationship.

It's been said that trust is the cornerstone in the foundation of any good relationship. It's possible that both of you may have developed major trust issues. First there is the ADD person who has not followed through with commitments and has made decisions that were impulsive, ultimately upsetting the equilibrium of the relationship. It makes sense that that kind of behavior would undermine their partner's trust. But the non-ADD person may also have some behaviors that undermine the trust of their ADD partner. These behaviors usually involve manipulation and control—manipulation of their partner, withholding information, and controlling their partner's behaviors and/or feelings. Granted, some of these controlling behaviors are a way to try and survive in the relationship. Unfortunately, those manipulative moves, although stemming from a need for survival, still undermine the trust of the ADD person. For the relationship to be a good one, you both need trust.

Learning to trust again may be difficult. This is why the issue of structure is so important for the person with ADD—we can use structure to help us be more trustworthy. If we give our word or commit to doing something, we need to follow through with that and make good on the commitment. Remember, first we must have a plan, and then work that plan regardless of how we feel. When we don't follow our plan, we set ourselves up for distrust. Then, when our partner doesn't trust us, we wonder why. Of course they don't trust us. We didn't do what we said we were going to do.

It's not that we're bad people. Our impulsiveness and poor follow-through set our partners up to distrust us. Work on improving your trustworthiness by using the structure we talked about earlier.

There is a huge movement across this country right now designed specifically to help men learn how to make good promises and how to make good on those promises. It is the Christian-based organization called Promise Keepers International. One of the core principles this organization teaches is the necessity of trustworthiness in healthy families and healthy relationships. It's important to our partner that when we give our word on something, they can count on us.

For the non-ADD partner, I want to validate the pain you've experienced. It's difficult being involved with someone who constantly changes their mind. I know that your trust has been challenged and that it may be difficult for you to trust at times. That makes sense. This is where we jump back to "easy does it."

I'm not asking you to trust when it feels inappropriate to trust or when trusting might hurt you more. I am suggesting that, as the two of you work together to create the successful romantic relationship you both want, at some point you'll have to put your trust on the line again. What will help is to learn as much as you can about ADD—what its characteristic behaviors are and how your partner is acting them out. Your partner is not trying to be a jerk. Chances are a lot of it is just ADD and some maladaptive behaviors that they have developed as a way to try to compensate for their disability.

Educating yourself about ADD, counseling, and a twelve-step group where you can safely vent your frustrations and develop supportive friendships—these are all powerful ways to learn how to cope with your partner's ADD without having to leave the relationship.

I remember an elderly lady telling me about her marriage of sixty-three years and describing some of the challenges she and her husband faced in their relationship. I asked her if she ever considered divorce. She replied, "No, I never did consider divorce—homicide was an option a couple of times, but never divorce." Kidding aside, if you love your partner and you want to make the relationship work, find an appropriate support network to help you through the rough spots.

If a breach of trust has so challenged your relationship that you feel like a ship cast upon the rocks, it's imperative that both of you get into counseling with a qualified therapist who knows and understands ADD in adults and who will help you work through those issues so you can both develop and build trust once again. This isn't always easy, but it's worthwhile. If you forego working through these issues now and leave your partner, chances are you will still have to work through some aspect of those issues later in life with your next partner.

Go see a therapist. Work the problem out together. Twelve-step groups are a great place to work through some of these issues on an individual basis. Pastoral counseling can often help. Usually medication for treatment of the ADD is a necessary tool for acquiring the ability to effectively address these issues. But wherever you go, you want people who will be supportive and encouraging. People who have a good understanding of what ADD is like in adults and how it affects romantic relationships. People who can help you work through these issues and help you develop trust again.

You can find those kinds of people through national support groups like the National Attention Deficit Disorder Association (ADDA). This organization is a resource of valuable information and also provides support groups for people who have ADD and non-ADD partners. Their national headquarters is located in Ohio, and you can reach them at (440) 350-9595. Their Website is www.add.org.

The oldest national organization committed specifically to educating about ADD in adults is the ADDult Information Exchange Network (ADDIEN) in Ann Arbor, Michigan. Their Website is www.addien.org, and their phone number is (734) 426-1659.

ChADD, which stands for Children and Adults with Attention Deficit Disorder is probably the largest organization for education and advocacy for people who have ADD. For more information contact their national office at (954) 587-3700, or visit their Website at www.chadd.org.

The national organizations listed above have a plethora of information to share about ADD. Each organization holds yearly international conferences that include the world's most authoritative experts in the realm of ADD.

Next in the Sweetheart Approach is the letter "H", which stands for HUMOR. Humor is important in relationships, *especially* when ADD is involved. Learn to laugh. Shared laughter makes life a lot more bearable and enjoyable. When you stop to think about it, some of the stuff that goes on because of our ADD *is* pretty funny.

Humor takes the pressure off. It makes it safe to make mistakes and to be human.

Look for the humor in all of this stuff. It's there. Use humor as a release valve for the pressure that can build up when you just can't get things right or when you make mistakes. This goes along with the concept of "easy does it." Take it easy on yourself and laugh. It's *okay* to be human. It's *okay* to make mistakes. It's *okay* to be imperfect. And it's *okay* to laugh about this stuff.

I once went to a workshop entitled "You're Taking This Life Thing Way Too Seriously." It was all about having fun. Remember, don't take this ADD thing too seriously. Don't get stuck worrying about whether you're getting this right or that right. Let go of it for awhile. Relax and have some fun. Laugh at it. Once the two of you know what's taking place neurobiologically in your brain, and that you may or may not have any control over some things, it makes it a lot easier to laugh.

All my life I've been in situations in which I was talking with someone I knew quite well, and for whatever reason I could not remember their name. The shame. The guilt. The embarrassment. The mental gymnastics I went through trying to cover up for not remembering their name. Fortunately, the woman I was dating at the time and who is now my wife had been learning a lot about ADD, and together we both started applying the Sweetheart Approach.

I'll never forget the day Terri and I were talking when all of a sudden, I went to address her by name and—for the life of me—I couldn't remember her name. Using the Sweetheart Approach— specifically the humor part—I just paused for a moment, and said, "Pardon me, what was your name again?" We both cracked up. My inability to recall Terri's name had nothing to do with my love or commitment to her as my partner; it only had to do with my ADD. When we know it's related to neurobiology, we can laugh about it instead of feeling shame and pain.

I have a toll-free number specifically for people to call and record their most embarrassing moment related to their ADD and how and why they were able to laugh about it. That number is (800) 555-9205, extension 5858. There are thousands and thousands of stories out there. You probably know some yourself. If you do, I'd love to hear from you—and please leave me your name and phone number so I can call you back.

Maybe you can't laugh about your ADD behaviors yet, but hang in there. Just remember, some of the stuff we do really *is* pretty funny. And if we can learn to laugh about it instead of taking it so personally, life becomes a lot easier.

The next concept in the Sweetheart Approach is ESTEEM. Hold each other in high regard. You're both unique and wonderful in your own special way, and you both deserve respect for your individualism. Your unique approaches to life can create a synergy in which your life together becomes better than either of you on your own. Use your differences to your collective advantage.

If you're upset with your partner and need to blow off some steam from time to time, go to a twelve-step meeting and unload. Or talk with your therapist about the stuff that's driving you nuts. These are healthy ways to release intense emotions and accumulated irritations. That's normal, and healthy. But it's quite a different thing if your energy is spent tearing down your partner, either to their face or behind their back. That's not going to help them and it's not going to help your relationship.

When we speak and think negatively about our partner it only reinforces our own negative beliefs and causes us to devalue our partner, not only in our eyes, but also in the eyes of others—friends, neighbors, and family. This devaluation is a kind of character assassination. Could anyone really expect their relationship to thrive and flourish when they constantly assassinate the character of their mate? Of course not. So if you find you're acting as the hit man in the character assassination of your mate, it's time to stop.

There's only one good way to talk about your partner behind their back—and I hope you'll do this. In fact, I implore you to do this. Instead of tearing your partner down, gossip regularly about their positive attributes. Speak highly of them. Focus on their strengths, and tell the world how wonderful they are in those areas. As you do this, *you* will develop a better opinion of your partner. You will begin to esteem them and recreate in your heart and mind respect for that which makes them special.

This doesn't mean that you esteem their bad behavior if their behavior is abhorrent. It does mean that you esteem the person and hold *them* in high regard.

I am convinced that an essential nutrient of life is to know that we are acceptable the way we are—that we are lovable with all of our flaws and good points. This doesn't mean that our dysfunctional behavior is lovable or acceptable, but it does mean that we as humans are. It's like the old adage: "You don't throw the baby out with the bath water." The "baby" in your romantic relationship deserves this same love, respect, and courtesy.

We all need to know we have value as humans if we're to have the courage to grow and develop to our greatest potential. Practice esteeming your partner and yourself so that you can both grow— and the relationship can grow.

There are only three basic concepts left in the Sweetheart Approach, and we're now up to the letter "A", which stands for ACCEPT. I believe it was Carl Rogers, the father of Person Centered Therapy, who once said, "Nothing can change until it becomes real." That is why the acceptance process is so important. Until we become willing to accept the reality of our ADD (or our partner's ADD), it's very difficult to move forward. Denial is not a bad thing. It is a self-protective mechanism we use to try to protect ourselves from pain. For whatever reason, some people need more protection from this kind of pain than others. You have to ask your-self, "Can accepting the reality of ADD be any worse than having the behavioral characteristics emanating from the ADD and not accepting its reality!"

So the first part of acceptance is to accept the reality of the ADD itself. The next step is to accept what you can and cannot change.

People cannot, by an act of their will, change the neurobiological functioning of their prefrontal cortex—the part of the brain from which classic ADD originates. If your prefrontal cortex isn't working right, you're not going to be able to change its functioning by wishing or hoping, no matter how bad you want it to change. This is why medication is so important in the treatment of ADD.

The Serenity Prayer has been used in twelve-step work for years to help teach acceptance:

> *God, grant me the serenity to accept the things I cannot change,*
> *the courage to change the things I can,*
> *and the wisdom to know the difference.*

The powerful words and message may be beneficial to you as a constant reminder that as humans, there are things we can't change—no matter how hard we try. What we need to do is to learn how to let go of those things so we can focus on the things we can change.

Whether it's the person with ADD having to learn how to accept their own limitations, or the partner of someone with ADD learning to accept their partner's disability, acceptance can take some time and it can sometimes be difficult. But acceptance is both necessary and possible. It helps to talk about the feelings you have about ADD with your partner, and with your therapist or in your support group. Talking about your feelings can be beneficial. Remember to talk with people who will be safe, supportive, and nurturing. That's why I encourage you to see a therapist who knows and understands ADD, or get involved in twelve-step work. Generally, therapists and twelve-step groups are safe.

Acceptance may take some time. That's okay. Remember to apply the Sweetheart Approach of "easy does it." Be gentle with yourself—and with your partner. This may be new territory for both of you. Allow yourselves time to adjust to the "label" of ADD. The more you know about ADD, the better-equipped you are to compensate for it—even capitalize on it. All of this will help in the acceptance process.

With acceptance comes freedom. Acceptance makes it easier to do some of the things we talked about earlier, such as being able to laugh about some of the crazy things we do, or being able to respect your partner in spite of their disability and some of the behaviors they exhibit from time to time. Acceptance makes these positive behaviors possible and makes life easier.

A friend of mine was extremely unhappy when he was first diagnosed with ADD. But the more Freddie talked about his unhappiness, the closer he came to acceptance of his ADD. He started educating himself about the characteristic behaviors associated with his type of ADD and the different parts of his brain that were involved. Not only did he reach acceptance, he went beyond that to celebration.

For the first time in his life, Freddie was finding answers to things he had struggled with for years. His life began to make more sense to him. He was able to better identify his strengths and weaknesses and to embrace the parts of his ADD which serve him marvelously, as well as accept the parts of his ADD that challenge him. He is better able to take care of himself by becoming more realistic about his abilities and expectations. This doesn't mean that everything turned up roses. It does mean that he avoided being upset and discouraged about his ADD and found out what he could do and what he couldn't do to make his life better.

Freddie had tremendous support from his wife during this process. She also educated herself about ADD and worked at understanding his perspective of life. He also worked at understanding her perspective—what being married to him must be like. They worked together as a team, and they've done really well. They have taken full advantage of the challenges they faced by using those challenges to create intimacy. Their love and respect for each other—coupled with help from their therapist and support group—made it possible for them to grow closer together and be even more loving towards each other.

That's not to say that they don't still face challenges. Life will always have plenty of challenges. But by facing the challenges together, they can continue to create intimacy. Their love is vibrant and alive because it is active rather than stagnant. What their relationship illustrates is the Sweetheart Approach in action.

Acceptance is the key that opens the door to healing, growth, and love.

The next letter is "R", and that stands for ROMANCE. Schedule romance into your lives. Make time for intimacy. It's easy to get caught up in the chaos of day-to-day living, so we frequently neglect this incredibly important area of our relationship.

Learn and practice the art of seducing your partner. Give and receive pleasurable, sensual touches. Find out what turns your partner on sexually. What turns your partner on may be very different from what gets you going. When you know what they like, do that for them (as long as it feels right for you too). Offer that as a gift to your mate—not because you have to, but because you love them.

If it's something you *have* to do, that's not love. Love is a choice. Find out what works for them and what works for you, and then express your gift of love in a way that works for both of you. There are many romantic (sexual and non-sexual) things you can do for your partner every day to enhance your relationship and keep the romance alive. Things like candlelit dinners, warming the car up for them on a cold winter morning, buying their favorite cologne, giving a quick therapeutic neck rub when times are stressful. Find out what makes them feel loved and minister to them. It's incredible what this can do for your relationship.

One of the things we know from neurobiological studies is that there are some very specific biochemical changes that take place in the brain when there is a release of endorphins associated with emotional and sexual intimacy. Emotional bonding is easier when endorphins are present. Talk about chemistry—it's real! So get your biochemistry sets out and get to work.

Regardless of what's going on in the relationship in terms of stress and tension and conflict, learn how to set that aside so the two of you can come together romantically. You both need intimate interactions with each other for bonding to take place.

If you don't want to be sexually intimate with your partner, that's something you need to talk about with them. If you can't talk about it with them one-on-one, then talk about it with the help of a counselor or therapist. Romantic love is supposed to be enjoyable. If it's not, then you need to see a physician who can assess what's taking place physically—to see if there is a physical problem which is causing the discomfort—or you need to see a therapist who can work with you on the emotional aspects of the sexual discomfort. Maybe you just need to sit down and talk with your partner and tell them what you need that you're not getting. Ask for what you want, and let them decide if that's a gift they want to give. Remember, love is a choice. You have the right to ask. They also have the right to decline.

The purpose of romantic and sexual intimacy in a relationship is to have a shared experience, and that shared experience needs to be enjoyable for both partners. Lack of good communication is one of the biggest obstacles to creating mutually satisfying intimacy. In a society which throws sex in our face on a daily basis in newspapers, magazines, books, television, and movies, it's amazing how afraid we are to really talk about sex. If talking about your sexual likes and dislikes or listening to your partner's sexual desires is a scary area for you to venture into, get some help from a professional. That's why we're here. Know that you are not alone in your fear of talking about sex. One of the reasons for all the sexual bravado coming from the media in the first place is that we are too afraid to talk appropriately and openly about sex. Our culture is terrified to talk about real intimacy. So take a deep breath and call your therapist or clergy and get some help.

Last but not least in the Sweetheart Approach is the letter "T", which stands for THANKFULNESS. Choose to focus on what the two of you have that you can be thankful for. Foster a sense of gratitude in your heart.

A study published in the summer of 1995 concluded that having an attitude of gratitude can actually change the biochemistry in our brains and ward off certain types of depression. For years, recovery programs have promoted the concept of having an "Attitude of Gratitude" because it is important to recovery. We now know that in terms of biochemistry, consciously changing the way you think—fostering an attitude of gratitude—can actually change the way you feel.

Focus on your partner's strengths instead of their weaknesses. Find what you can be thankful for in regard to the ADD component of your relationship—and what you can be thankful for in general. A grateful heart is a salve that heals the relationship. Gratitude does not deny reality; it chooses to focus on that which will bring healing and encouragement.

I know in my own life, when I hyperfocus on "the bad stuff" and stay stuck in a negative thought process, I feel terrible, emotionally and physically. When I change my focus to something I can be thankful for—in spite of the bad stuff—something changes inside of me, and I begin to feel better. This experience is a natural phenomenon that's related to the biochemical changes in my brain that occur as a result of choosing to think about things to be thankful for. This is not just some pie-in-the-sky idea in a textbook, it's something that really does work to change the way we feel.

Discover the benefits of putting STRUCTURE in your life, and

WELCOME the differences between you and your partner. ENCOURAGE each other. Be gentle with each other—EASY DOES IT. TRUST and be trustworthy in your behaviors and your actions. Use HUMOR to laugh at the silly things you do that are the result of ADD. ESTEEM yourself and your partner. ACCEPT what is reality and what you can and can't change. Use ROMANCE as a way to stay connected and increase the bonding between the two of you. Practice THANKFULNESS for what you've got and for what you are learning.

Regardless of whether you are ever diagnosed as having ADD, regardless of whether you ever take any sort of medication for ADD, the concepts and principles presented in the Sweetheart Approach will have a tremendous impact on your relationship and in your life if you use them.

To help you remember to use the Sweetheart Approach, photocopy this page and put it on your car's dashboard. Tape it to the mirror in the bathroom. Attach it to the refrigerator. Carry it in your pocket. Keep it as a handy reminder of ten things you can do on a daily basis to energize your relationship.

THE SWEETHEART APPROACH

STRUCTURE
WELCOME
ENCOURAGE
EASY Does It
TRUST
HUMOR
ESTEEM
ACCEPT
ROMANCE
THANKFULNESS

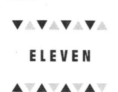

ELEVEN

Fifty Ways to Keep Your Lover

Now that you have a better understanding of ADD and a new appreciation of your partner, you're champing at the bit to move on to the next step—adding even more love and spice to your relationship. Great idea. Use this list as an inspiration to jump-start your own creative juices.

Trust me—you *can* be wildly successful in your romance.

1. Go on a date together each week. One week you plan it, the next week your partner plans it. Trade off each week so you share the responsibility. Be creative. Have fun.

2. Hide little hand-written love notes in each other's billfold, pocket, purse, car . . . anywhere your lover will accidentally come across them each day. Also, hide them in places they will only come across once in a while. You'll forget where you hid them, and when your lover finds them, you'll be as pleasantly surprised as they are.

3. Plan a weekend alone together at a romantic, secluded place like the mountains or the beach. Stay in the honeymoon suite at a quaint little bed-and-breakfast.

4. Make a surprise romantic dinner at home and serve it in the bedroom with candles, soft music—and no phones or pagers on or nearby.

5. Take your medication religiously, as prescribed.

6. Give your lover a gift certificate for a full-body massage.

7. Thank your partner out of the blue for something nice they did for you. Maybe just for even loving you, since they make your life more complete. Surprises and appreciation make your partner feel loved.

8. Take a bath together. Soft lights. Soft music. Soft sighs.

9. Work at resolving conflicts only at times when your prescribed ADD medications are in your body. Conflict resolution will be easier when your brains are working right.

10. Send flowers, balloons, or something special for no special reason.

11. Dedicate a song to your partner on their favorite radio station at a time when you know they'll be listening.

12. It's never too late to say you're sorry.

13. Breakfast in bed . . . with dessert afterwards.

14. Go to couples counseling . . . even if everything is great.

15. If your partner is stressed out about work or some other stressful situation, take them on a surprise picnic to a place they would enjoy—a park bench, in front of a fountain, or at an art gallery . . . someplace where they can relax into you and away from the stress.

16. Wash your partner's hair for them. Purchase special shampoo and conditioner to use just for this occasion.

17. Personally give your partner a pedicure—everything, the works.

18. Try new and different ways to make your lovemaking more sensual and enjoyable. Edible massage oils. Flower petals strewn on the sheets. Satin sheets.

19. Surprise your partner with something they love but you really don't care too much for. For example, take her to the opera (if that's what she likes) even if you only like country-western music. Do it with no strings attached and without a hint of complaining.

20. When conversations become angry, before they become too angry, take a break and come back later to solve the problem.

21. Agree that if and when there is ever going to be a huge argument, you both have to get naked for the argument.

22. Feed each other Chinese food with chopsticks while sitting together in a nice warm bath. You cannot feed yourself. You have to feed each other.

23. Set aside some time each week to discuss with your mate the positive and negative aspects of that week. You can talk about anything—work, family, the relationship—but set this time aside to listen and talk with your partner.

24. Give your partner a gift certificate for housecleaning.

25. Let go of things that are not that important to you, and negotiate with as much zeal for what your partner wants as you do for what you want.

26. Take something you both enjoy the taste of and dab little bits of it on each other's body to taste and nibble off in most enjoyable ways.

27. After a sensuous shower together, give each other a full-body massage. Have the room lit with candles. Play soft music. And do not make love until both of you have had your massage. If you fail at this step, start the process all over again.

28. Spend time together each week without the TV on, radios playing, kids interrupting, or magazines to read. Just sit there or lay there and be with each other.

29. Surprise your lover by doing the household chores they usually do.

30. Ask your partner to tell you what they would like to do differently when the two of you make love next time.

31. Have your partner's car washed and waxed for them.

32. Send your partner a surprise E-mail.

33. If your partner goes out of town on a trip, hide a greeting card for each day of the week in their luggage.

34. Discover something you both enjoy and do it often.

35. Out of the blue, take your partner out of the city and away for the day. Or if you live in the country, take them into the city for the day.

36. Play strip poker with each other.

37. Make love in a different place other than just your bed. Try a walk-in closet. On the bathroom floor. In the kitchen on the counter. The back seat of your car.

38. If you're going on a long trip by car, secretly plan a special lunch, or a treat, or a special romantic song on tape—something that you know your partner will enjoy.

39. Go see a romantic movie together.

40. Take your partner to a surprise vacation spot—someplace they have always wanted to go, but have never been.

41. Usually in a relationship, one partner is more verbal than the other. If that's you, resist talking sometimes in order to create a quiet space in which your lover can communicate.

42. Go on a couples retreat to learn more about each other.

43. Find a Bible and read 1 Corinthians 13 (the love chapter) together.

44. Let go of having to have the last word.

45. Rather than argue your point, try to really listen and not only understand what your partner's point is, but also why it is so important to them.

46. Together, volunteer to serve a Thanksgiving day meal at the local homeless shelter.

47. Buy a sexy and romantic game the two of you could play together.

48. Tell your lover a bedtime story. It may be something you make up. It may be sexy, romantic, funny, or just plain silly. If you've got a lot of courage, act out the story as a play at the foot of the bed with you as the only actor.

49. Out of nowhere, take five minutes to tell your partner as many things as you can that you love, appreciate, and admire about them.

50. Do something outlandishly romantic like a hot air balloon ride, or sailing or soaring, or a train trip complete with private deluxe room in the sleeper car.

Find out what your partner likes and do that for them. Let them know what you like. Take a pro-active stance in nurturing the love that you share. Some of the things on your list can and probably need to be serious. But there probably needs to be a lot more fun things on your list in order to keep the love alive. Remember the things you've learned in this book. Go back and re-read it. If you didn't the first time through, underline things that strike your fancy as being important, and then use those things as a springboard to write your own list. This is not just a project you are going to be working on for the next couple of weeks. Together, you are creating tools that can and will last a lifetime, tools that will help keep your love energized and your relationship romantic.